DUDE, I'M JUST A GIRAFFE

A MEMOIR BY CHRIS STUART

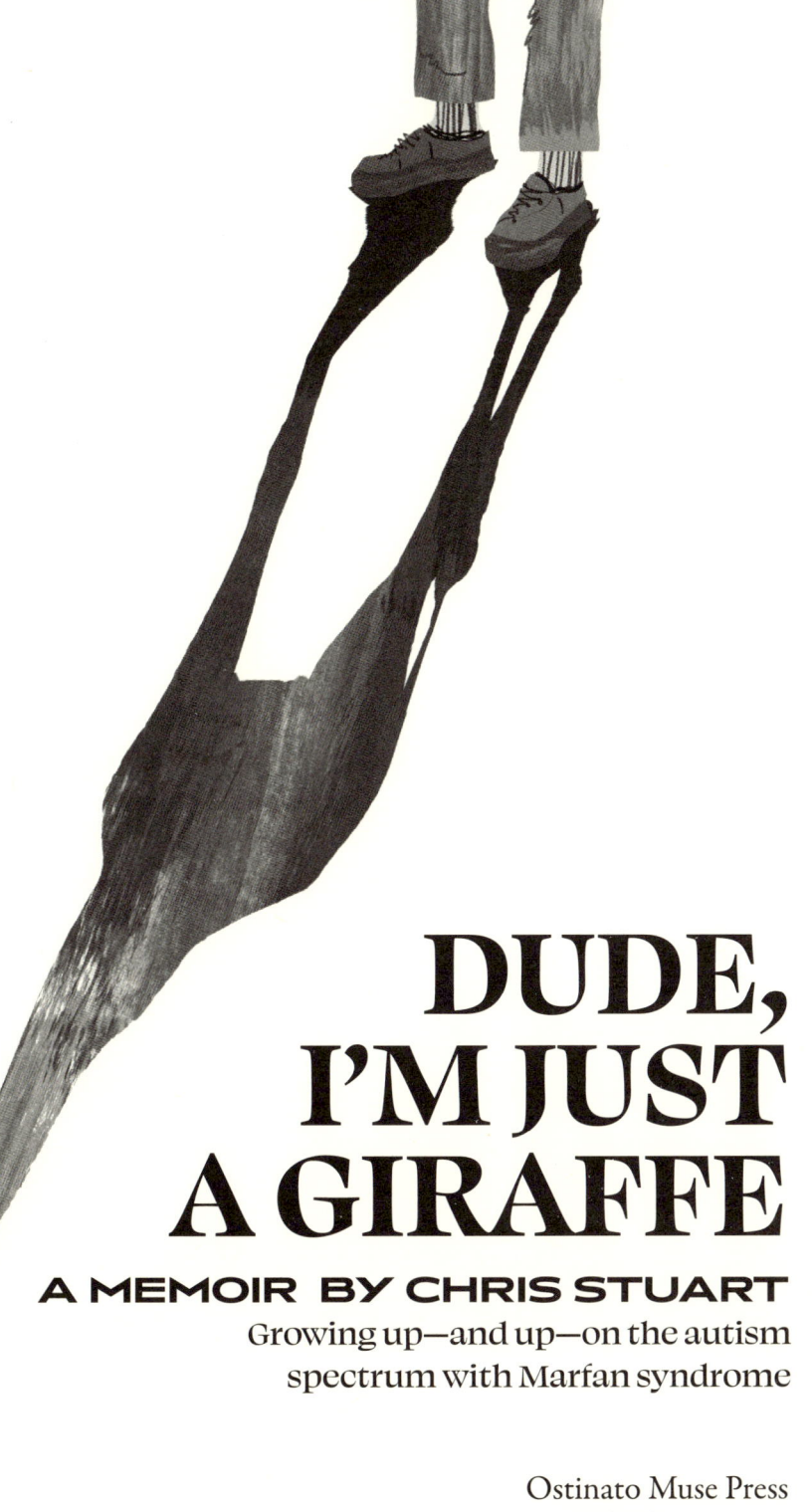

DUDE, I'M JUST A GIRAFFE

A MEMOIR BY CHRIS STUART

Growing up—and up—on the autism spectrum with Marfan syndrome

Ostinato Muse Press
Nashville, Tennessee

Copyright 2021 ©

Chris Stuart

All rights reserved

Book Design by Benjamin Rumble

Typeface is Garamond Premier Pro

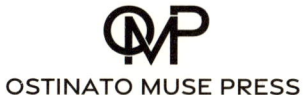

OSTINATO MUSE PRESS

1	INTRODUCTION
3	ACKNOWLEDGMENTS
5	PREFACE
9	CHAPTER ONE: MARFAN HAPPENS
21	CHAPTER TWO: A TALL GIRAFFE
35	CHAPTER THREE: ARIZONA BOUND
41	CHAPTER FOUR: LIMITATIONS

57 CHAPTER FIVE:
TRANSITIONS

67 CHAPTER SIX:
IS THIS MY LIFE?

79 CHAPTER SEVEN:
OPERATIONS DU JOUR

91 CHAPTER EIGHT:
NEVER-ENDING CHANGES

103 CHAPTER NINE:
PISSING OFF THE GIRAFFE

113 CHAPTER TEN:
GETTING IT TOGETHER

123 DEDICATIONS

THIS BOOK IS DEDICATED
TO MY MOTHER

ANN REINKING

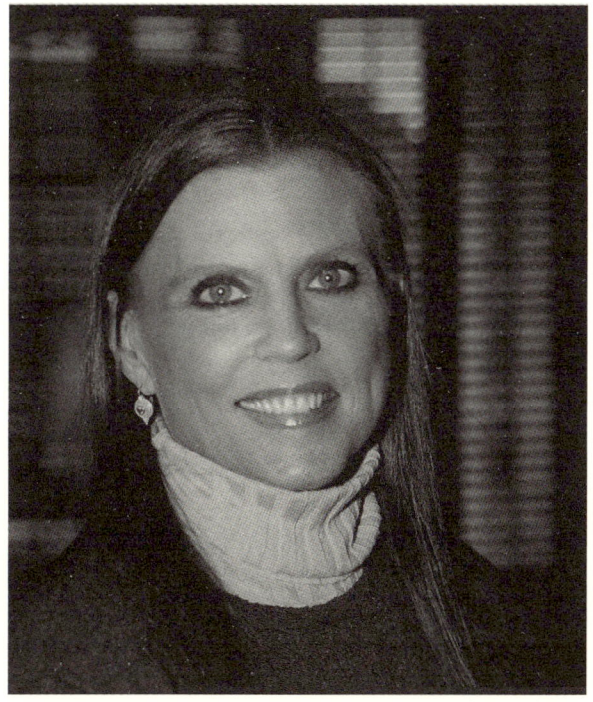

photo by Brenda Siemer

INTRODUCTION

I'm just blown away by this book. I'm not sure anyone will truly believe all that Chris has been through and endured throughout his lifetime.

That's the truth about Marfan. You just never know what is going to hit you and, it sounds cliché to say this, but "rolling with the punches" is all you can do, and no one is doing it better than Chris! He has endured more than most and also has his emotional challenges to deal with...being on the spectrum with autism. But through it all, he studied, graduated, built his relationships, and his friendships, both young and old, and knew how to surround himself with people who only made him better! And he did it on his own, and he did it his way.

I'm amazed at how together and articulate this young man is, regardless of his physical and emotional challenges. He is stronger than us all and amazingly self-aware. That was the one shocker in the entire book -- that through it all he was so expressive, sharp, and spot on.

I wish I could hug Annie right now and tell her what an amazing son she has and how appreciated she is. There is no one who felt more empathy than she did for her son and the Marfan community. She gave so much and will be remembered and cherished always. Chris, you have your mom's heart and soul and know that she is resting in peace just knowing how you deal with all the challenges that come your way!

Congratulations! Such a good read.

Karen Murray
Board of Directors
The Marfan Foundation

ACKNOWL-
EDGMENTS

I'd first like to, as cliché as it may be, thank my parents. Both step and biological. Ann Reinking, Peter Talbert, and James Stuart. After all, I wouldn't exist as I am today, both literally and figuratively, without them. I hope you can read this wherever you are, mom.

Secondly, I would like to thank the Marfan Foundation, and in particular Eileen Masciale, for quite literally dropping this opportunity onto my lap. I am forever grateful!

Thirdly, I would like to thank Patricia Tusay for being my editor and general taskmaster. At times I know it must have felt like we were teacher and student again and you were making sure I did my homework at times, instead of the professional relationship editor and author should have. But without you, this volume would not exist, so my eternal gratitude is yours! As well as my eternal apologies!

Fourth, I'd like to thank my roommates, Liz Foldi and Barbara Sause, who had to live with me through all of this.

Lastly, I wish to thank everyone I interviewed for this project. That includes everyone already named besides Masciale, but also: Eileen Masciale, Thomas Fisher, Dr. Dietz, Dr. Sponseller, Julie, Robert Erdman, John Greer, and my sister Maren Stuart!

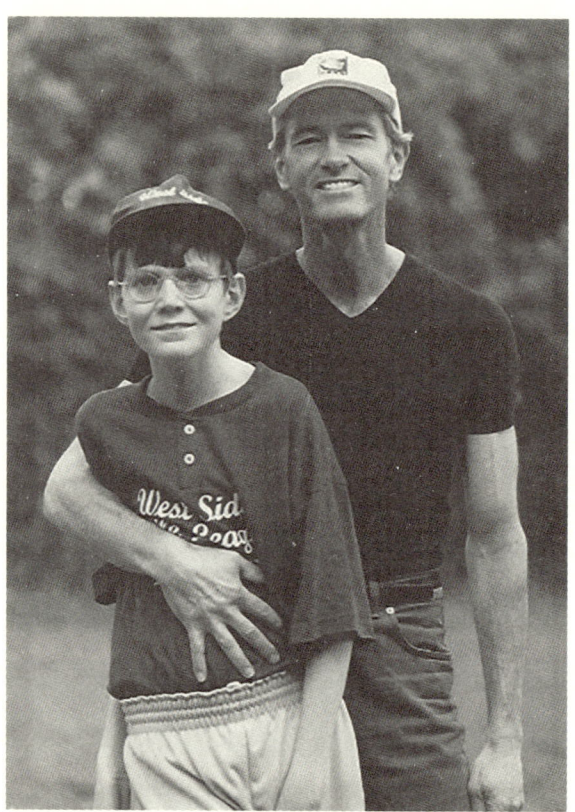

With my Dad at a T-ball game when I still lived in New York City. I also played soccer and basketball until my heart operations and back surgery made sports impossible.

PREFACE
BY PETER TALBERT

With many emotional and physical ups and downs Chris came into my life when he was a little more than two years old. He had no words—at least no decipherable English words. He spoke his own language, made up of various sounds, which seemed to be as highly descriptive of his thoughts, moods and emotions as any in the world, (if only we had the Rosetta Stone to decipher it). Owing to his autism, he would not start adding real English words into the mix until he was five, at which point every week saw an ever-expanding universe of words and phrases being used. In the coming years, we were also coming to terms with his Marfan with overwhelming odds and trying situations.

Now, some thirty years later, he has graduated from Arizona State University with a degree in English despite missing close to five years of school time because of hospitalizations and recovery times; multiple interstices that have severely restricted his physical world. He has persevered over every obstacle that Mother Nature and the universe has thrown at him.

He is funny, outgoing, endlessly inquisitive, and can argue a bump off a log. He does not so much think outside the box as needs to occasionally find the box to reign in his incredible imagination. When I have asked myself the question "Were it in my ability, would I wish away the Marfan and the autism?" "Of course," I think. I would give anything to save Chris from the physical agonies he has endured over the years, and the stigma that accrues to anyone who presents differently in speech, personality, and thought. If he had not been galvanized and heat pressured like a diamond by the unusual internal/external forces in his life, who would he be today? The young man I would not give up for anything, Chris, is without a doubt the single bravest and strongest man I have known in my life. I marvel at his humor and resilience. He is an inspiration to me and my wife. I believe he will be just such an inspiration for other kids with Marfan and their parents. He is my hero, and I am immeasurably proud of him and his first book.

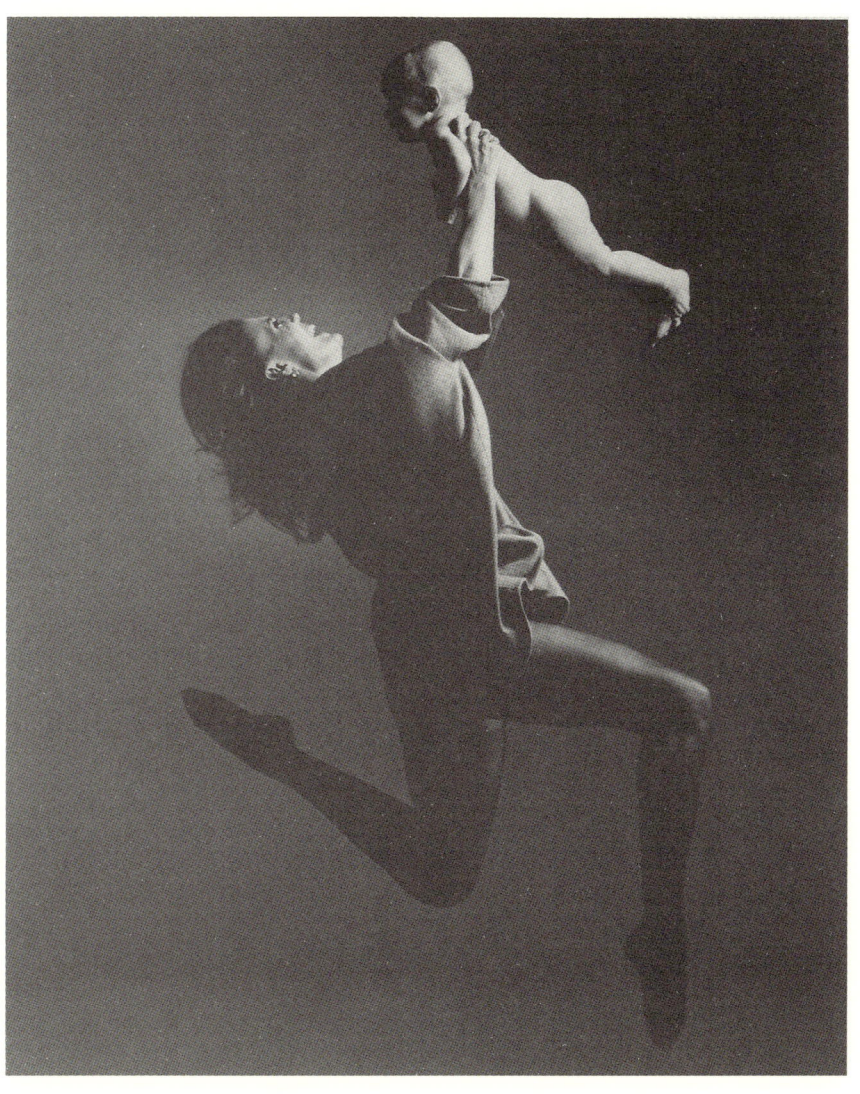

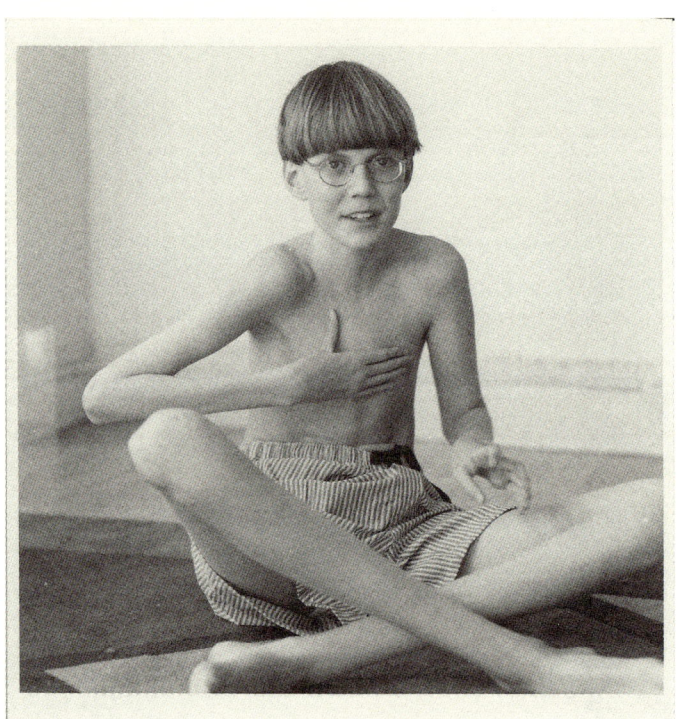

Showing the long limbs associated with Marfan in one of a series of remarkable photos taken by photographer Rick Guidotti.

CHAPTER ONE: MARFAN HAPPENS

Let us start this thing from the very beginning. Once, there was an eternal void—an actual void. Not a vacuum, a void; nothing, no existence. Then, there was light, matter, and expansion. Plasma becomes space, becomes stars, becomes planets, becomes water, and becomes single celled life, and then... millions of years of evolution! This resulted in humans; Mom and Dad meet and then—I was the result. Obviously, the whole point of all this is that I am the ultimate end point of fourteen billion years of existence. I mean, of course I am! Why else do you think this all happened? If you have not figured it out by now, my writing style is a bit flippant, and perhaps attributed to my ADHD and combined with my own creativity! Either way, I have evolved into this type of a writer. To be honest, I love it. In other words, I go with the flow in writing as I do with my life.

So yes, my birth happened. I decided to start here because, well, I started here. This is when I got Marfan syndrome and autism. In the case of my autism, it may be genetic. I also have a bit of a yarn to spin for you about my birth. This was conveyed to me by my mother after the fact and not from memory for obvious reasons, and I believe it will adequately establish pertinent details about myself and my coping mechanisms.

So, on the ninth day of January 1990 AD (or CE), I was born in a hospital in the Floridian city of Clearwater. I did not stay in Florida long and, therefore, I will not be mentioning Florida a great deal or much at all really. I was about two-and-a-half when I moved to New York City. I did not get my official Marfan diagnosis until I was six; however, my mother had deep suspicions that I had this earlier. She moved back to New York with me to be closer to specialists. Therefore, I feel comfortable starting here; it was not long after this pivotal point in my history of the universe that Marfan started affecting my life.

According to my mom, instead of crying right out of the birth canal like any sane baby would, I apparently came out as silent as a lamb. I then looked side to side and further surveyed the room with dawning horror upon my infant face. Unlike all the other babies, I had to be sure that I was indeed totally and thoroughly up a particular creek before I made my complaint to the universe for putting me in this crummy situation soon to unfold. Once I had confirmed that I did indeed exist and that, yes, it was indeed all downhill from here, only then did I act like a normal baby and complain to the manager of this and every establishment to follow.

As this is not a full-on autobiography, I am limiting my beginning existence to my experiences growing up and living with and, most importantly, coping with Marfan syndrome. Besides, there really isn't much in the way of stories I know about my life between my birth and my tentative diagnoses, and I have little desire to intrude into whatever marital issues that led to my biological parents' divorce. However, I do have an older half-sister and she had her own thoughts of seeing my struggle as I continued to grow:

> Something that is deeply engrained in me is that family is number one. Chris and I only lived together for just over two years. Yet from the day I laid eyes on him, when he was in the hospital as a newborn, I instantly felt a connection. It was my first time being a sister. I did not know how it was going to develop as we have an 11 year age gap and we lived in different states most of our lives. But throughout the years, I have felt an undying love and loyalty to always be there for him. As for his health conditions, it didn't change any way I felt about him... The key thing for me as an older sister is that I want to help protect and make sure he is never in pain or if/when he needs help, I am there. It was not easy seeing him through several of the larger surgeries (two heart, one back and ankle). It was hard not being able to do anything to make the pain go away. I really look up to my brother and how he handled every procedure with little to no complaints. I remember after one heart surgery, they offered him some major pain killers and all he wanted was *Advil*. He is a champ. I really look up to Chris (literally and figuratively). I would not want any other brother any other way! (Maren Stuart)

I must agree with Maren, family is everything. She has been there for me right from the beginning.

I was about two-and-a-half when my mom took me to the Yale New Haven Center, for what I do not really know. Mom does not really recall the exact reason either, as it was about three decades ago. However, it was probably for a general "check to see if your new infant is healthy and doesn't have some terminal illness" checkup. After all, I was properly diagnosed with high functioning autism at this point, so we were there for more than just cardiology. While there, a Doctor Linda (as I shall refer to her) told my mom that she was probably right about my having Marfan syndrome. You see, my mom was something of a fan of President Lincoln, and knew he had Marfan syndrome or at least was suspected to have had the condition. So, let us have my mom explain:

> Oh well, when you were born, I noticed how long your fingers and toes were! Of course, back then I just said you were going to be a pianist or basketball player or something like that. Then, when you were somewhere around two, I think, yes, two, I started noticing developmental things for your high functioning autism. So, I went to an expert about that; Dr. Linda Maze, and she's the one who had said that not only are you a functioning autistic but you had Marfan syndrome.
>
> She suspected you had Marfan and, by that time, I kind of did too because you were taller than any of the other kids your age. I knew you just had it. Big Lincoln fan girl here and I happen to know about Abraham Lincoln having Marfan because as you know, I love Lincoln. I read an article in either *Time* or *Newsweek* that spoke about Marfan syndrome and that Abraham Lincoln may have had it. (Ann Reinking)

And there you have it right from my mom, that I was informed that I looked just like what our dear dead forefather looked like while young, having some of the same physical features.

Unfortunately, while very accomplished and highly respected from what I have heard, this doctor was not qualified enough to make a proper diagnosis. And so, we followed this up by going to another so-called expert. Details here are unfortunately a bit scarce, mostly because Mom said she forgot a lot about this man in disgust. She does not even remember the man's name. After all, he, a supposed expert, said I did not in fact have Marfan syndrome. He was very confident and arrogant in this diagnosis as well. He knew that I did not have the condition. I will tell you right now that I have scars from all the surgeries that prove him wrong, but if Mom was more trusting in this situation with this man, there is a very good chance I would have died of an aneurysm at a very young age. Thank goodness my mom persisted, as she was not happy with the diagnosis and noticed other things were going on with me. At this point, her emotions were driving her to get a complete diagnosis:

> You are always glad to have a diagnosis even if you already know there is something not right, that you were different. She suspected, that

is Dr. Maze suspected you had it by two-and-a-half. This was by the time you were getting other things, such as you had suddenly gone myopic, that is nearsighted. Do you remember how suddenly you could not see the chalkboard? Then your dentist said that you have a very high palate. Then I think it hit home when a bunch of symptoms popped up, just your general look, you were lanky, you were taller than anybody you know, and your wrist started taking on a shape that was very Marfan like. You certainly noticed it when you got the diagnosis how your hands sitting in your wrists were a little different from the rest and just the general construct of your body. When you were six, I asked your pediatrician where I should go to get a proper diagnosis because he felt that it was Marfan as well. He thought he heard a murmur or something in your heart, but I cannot quite remember. He gave us an answer and we went to Dr. Steinfeld located in Mt Sinai Hospital. There it was in black and white—on paper, no wiggle room anymore—and I could not say you are going to be a pianist. I could not say you are going to be a great basketball player and I was pretty sure by then, but now it was definite. So yes, I was sad in the beginning. You do not want your child to have any issues or challenges. However, I would never give up on you. Your doctor was the one who said—I think his name was also Christopher—we could get in with Dr. Hal Dietz in Baltimore as that would be the best place for you. This would be at Johns Hopkins, a hospital in Baltimore. Dietz and Steinfeld both saw that you had an enlargement in your ascending aorta, in the root, and so then we just would have a yearly checkup when you had your echocardiogram. (Ann Reinking)

So, there I was, six years old when it happened. I was given this confirmation by Dr. Steinfeld at Mt. Sinai Hospital and I am sure I was informed. However, if I was, I do not really remember it that well. I really do not have any excuse this time for not remembering, as I was six, not two, and this was a significant event in my life. But then, there was a pretty good chance that I did not really register this visit as anything else other than another doctor visit and I was just bored. I am beginning to think that this is where some of my coping mechanisms started to kick in. I may have feigned boredom, acted bored or tuned out as a defense mechanism. I am also pretty sure we were all already operating under the auspices that I had the condition; this was just a final confirmation. I do not really remember a life without some knowledge of having issues with my heart. I do remember either not really understanding the critical component of it at that point or ignoring most of it.

The fact that the condition would not really affect me directly for a few more years, may have contributed to my lack of full comprehension of Marfan in general. However, this confirmation, while likely something of a formality for me and my immediate family (which by that point would include my stepfather, Peter Talbert), if an admittedly needed one to receive proper medical treatment, was anything but a mere formality for two other members of my extended family. You see, once this confirmation/diagnosis occurred, the entirety of my still-living blood relatives were asked to come in for similar screenings. According to the doctor who was there from the beginning for us, overseeing every aspect of my care was Dr. Dietz from Johns Hopkins:

> Marfan syndrome is a disorder of the connective tissue, the material between the cells that give tissues form and strength. The connective tissue also provides cues to neighboring cells regarding how they should behave. In Marfan syndrome there is a deficiency of a specific connective tissue protein called fibrillin-1. This causes a predictable set of features in many parts of the body including the heart, blood vessels, skeleton and eye. People with Marfan syndrome have bones that grow excessively, causing tall stature with particularly long arms, legs, fingers, and ribs. Elongation of the ribs can cause the chest wall to protrude outward or to indent inward. Other skeletal features include loose joints, flat feet, and curvature of the spine. The heart can show floppiness and leakage of heart valves. This can cause strain on the heart muscle if not recognized and treated. The most serious complication of Marfan syndrome is enlargement of the aorta, the major blood vessel carrying blood away from the heart. There is particular risk for enlargement of the base of the aorta, called the aortic root. If this area becomes too large, there is a risk of aortic tear or rupture. Other regions of the aorta and other blood vessels can show enlargement and tear in Marfan syndrome. The eye can show dislocation of the eye lens, which normally sits in the center of the eye and is required to focus light properly. The eye can also show excessive growth, causing nearsightedness. Other rarer eye complications include detachment of the nerve layer in the back of the eye called the retina or high eye pressure called glaucoma. Chris has shown many of these complications of Marfan syndrome and has required surgical intervention for aortic enlargement, aortic tear, and curvature of the spine. (Dr. Dietz)

Because this is known as a genetic condition, and thus inheritable, there was a fair chance that I was not the only one in my family who had the condition. As it turned out, I was the only one in my family to have this condition. It was decided that my Marfan was not inherited at all but was the result of a spontaneous mutation. I was not, however, the only one in my family with a life-threatening heart condition. My biological father was found to have been on the verge of multiple aneurysms and required immediate surgery:

> In 1999, Chris was diagnosed with Marfan syndrome. This means I had to go in [to Johns Hopkins] to get checked [for Marfan syndrome]. So, I went in and had a meeting with Dr. Hal Deitz, who ordered a sonogram done on my ascending aorta. I remember [Deitz] coming back out from another room, and he said, "I have good news and I have bad news." So, I asked him to give me the good news first. Deitz responded, "The good news is that you do not have Marfan syndrome. The bad news is that you have an identical degenerative aortic aneurysm that seems to be just like the condition your son has, but luckily is not. However, you are already in the range where you need surgery, so you best get [the surgery] done, or you'll be asleep for a long time." This was in March of 1999, and I came in for surgery mid-September of the same year. Dr. Deitz took care of me during my recovery time, and for several years after. He has told me that if I had not had this intervention when I did, I might not still be here. For this, I have a deep sense of gratitude towards my son Chris for getting his diagnosis which forced me to get checked, thus discovering that I had this degenerative disease. (Jim Stuart)

My cousin Jacob, from my mother's side of the family, was also found to have a predisposition towards developing aneurysms. I do believe they thought he had Marfan syndrome as well for a bit there, as I remember conversations with him that said as much, but in the end, his condition was different. He still required a bevy of surgeries later in life, just as I did, and this was a bonding experience for the two of us. These two people, both very important to me, would almost certainly be dead if I had not gotten my diagnosis.

It should be noted that, before I actually started to undergo surgeries in response to the condition, Marfan syndrome really did not change my life beyond the need to take a regimen of pills every evening and morning. Yes, there was the fact that I could not participate in any contact sport, but back then I really could not have cared less. I was not exactly sedentary; I had too much nervous energy for that. However, most of my interests were sedentary, such as video games, anime, and cartoons (though at that age, I didn't really know that distinction; they were all comics). Reading would come later in life, and so would the Internet. The long and short of the matter was that until I had to go under the knife, all Marfan syndrome was to me was a new set of pills to ingest. So, let us move on to when I had to go under the knife.

Would you call me a liar if I said was excited for my first surgery? For one, I was too young to truly understand the concept that I could potentially die while in surgery. Yes, for a surgery like this, that chance is beyond remote, but it still likely adds to the anxiety of anyone who would undergo surgery for the first time while being sufficiently old enough to actually understand the concept of death. I was too busy for the Grim Reaper.

To be honest, my only real prior experience with the idea of surgery was in the form of cartoons and video games. Surgery turned *John 117* into the *SPARTAN-II* super soldier *Master Chief*, peerless defender of the human race against a horde of alien zealots. Surgery made *Inspector Gadget* into the Swiss army knife of people. *The Six Million Dollar Man* was named for his six-million-dollar surgery. I had a very childish and unrealistic notion of surgery back then. In retrospect, it certainly was to my advantage even if it was my reality.

Perhaps the main reason for my innocent and naive excitement was novelty. I was a child addicted to novelty. As an example, I gave up delicious, packed lunches in order to see what school cafeteria food tasted like. Coping with the unknown was kind of like going headlong into new experiences for the sake of the experience. Yep, I was that kid.

To be fair to my twelve-year-old self, this was my first heart surgery and by far the least draining of all my surgeries. Strange to say that about a procedure that involved my heart, that it did not strike me as a serious blow, but it is true, and I will go into further details later. I wish to stay in somewhat chronological order with regards to all my procedures. As to the details, it is time to fill in those gaps.

The procedure was done at Johns Hopkins Hospital. (This is the research branch of Johns Hopkins School of Medicine, the medical arm of Johns Hopkins University). I was quite surprised to find out that I was technically being operated on in a school environment, but university grounds or not, Johns Hopkins Hospital is one of the best in the world and is the leader in Marfan research. I am not sure I was aware of all the distinctions at the time as I was too busy concentrating on my novel experience.

The hospital is based in Baltimore, in the state of Maryland. I admit, despite commuting there every June for my regular checkup, my knowledge of the state and city are somewhat limited beyond a few select locales. The area around the hospital and the bay has all the hotels and higher-end restaurants and establishments. Then again, I was going there for medical reasons, not for pleasure. So, my limited knowledge is to be forgiven. I was young and had my own agenda.

As for more details, it was Dr. Duke Cameron who performed my first open heart surgery upon my ascending aorta. He replaced my dangerously inflated ascending aorta. This inflated area, pushing ever closer to a deadly aneurysm and/or full-on rupture, was removed and replaced with an artificial (though not mechanical; no pacemaker in me) graft.

We arrived a few days before the actual date of the procedure. My mom, both my dads (though Jim made his own arrangements; I stayed with Mom and Peter), two of my nannies, Beatrice and Lillian, and I believe some of my extended family and I stayed in one of the local hotels. We spent a few days vacationing and doing things such as going to tourist traps and nice restaurants and ordering over-priced room service. Baltimore cuisine is absolutely dominated by crab. I was not quite sure what my emotions were supposed to be at this point as I was on vacation. Then, the date of my procedure came. You can tell by now my priorities had little to do with my upcoming surgery. However, my mom was dealing with her son and his life-threatening surgery:

> How did I cope with all the medial procedures? Once again it was a learning curve. You know, in the beginning it's scary and tenuous because you don't really know, since you're new to it—a novice! Sometimes it was fascinating and sometimes I was afraid I was going to miss something. You know it is trying not to be overwhelmed. So yeah cover all your bases, but do not get overwhelmed because it is not going to do any good now. Try to stay cool and learn along the way. You are in good hands and that counts a lot emotionally and psychologically. But yeah, we were learning on the job. (Ann Reinking)

Mom took a very educational approach. I am sure this was the coping mechanism she was using, learning along the way.

Once we arrived at Johns Hopkins, and were herded to a very metallic room. Mechanical, as if they were planning on building war-machines in there instead of prepping an eleven-year-old for surgery. High-quality war-machines though; the place was clean and organized and very professional, like a research and development laboratory and not some dirty factory assembly line. But that did not change the fact that the place put mechanical efficiency over comforting its patients, something that was left to the human doctors. It seems that standards have changed somewhat since then, as while this won't be my last memory of a medical room prioritizing function over form (as it should; I want to live after this, not feel comfortable while dying), I haven't been met by such a room since.

You might be thinking I am telling you all of this to share with you some of my trauma. This poor child of eleven, who was about to undergo serious heart surgery, was greeted by this room out of cynical science fiction on the inhumanity of man. The sort of room better suited to birthing Robocop or Darth Vader, and not for starting the anesthesia routine needed to begin a life-saving operation for a pre-teen. Traumatic, it was not.

In fact, the eleven-year-old me thought it looked really cool. I had a strange, inexperienced notion of surgery after all, and Darth Vader and Robocop were childhood heroes of mine. But more importantly, I am pretty sure I just let the negative connotations of it all wash over me like a seawall against a wave. It is how I tend to deal with my problems, as you will see as we continue; I endure while focusing not so much on the positive but rather the pleasant. To latch onto pleasure, however fleeting, and push pain aside, however chronic, I was dealing my way. I am sure my parents and the others who came along with me were a lot more negatively impacted by this mechanical environment, considering what I was about to undergo.

Luckily for all it seemed, the anesthesiologist who was responsible for me provided the human touch we all needed. Even as unaffected as I was by it all, if my doctor's bedside manner had been bad, I would have been a lot more nervous. He even fielded my childish jokes about cyborgs and zombies. I had some idea that I could die during the procedure, but as the weird child that I was, my notion of death was colored by pop culture and cartoons, zombies and Chinese gods willing to train the souls of dead martial artists to be defenders of the universe. This was all very assuring to me.

I am uncertain what exactly the modern policy for anesthesiology for preteens and toddlers is, but back when I had my first surgery, those who were too young were given what my parents and I called a "potion" that prepped me for the proper anesthetic. I do not remember too much of anything at all after I ingested this potion, but the stories I heard said I was something of a cartoon character while I was being transported to the operating room. Apparently, I spent ten minutes in complete awe of my massive feet. I do remember what I said immediately before drinking it though. The anesthesiologist wished me good luck on my surgery. A standard pleasantry if ever there was one. Yes, I had a response. I always have a response!

I heard off in the distance something odd. "Good luck!" "But why would I need good luck?" I said. "I'm just going to sleep. You are the ones performing the surgery. You are the ones who need the luck."

Obviously, this is being remembered through the lens of my adult mind, English major extraordinaire, as I doubt I was quite that eloquent at eleven. Either way, this got everyone in the room laughing, with a nervous but relieved tint in retrospect. While this may have cut through the tension of the room, it also reminded everyone that there was a non-zero chance that I would end up dead by the end of the day a low chance yes, but still non-zero in my mind. My coping skills already decided I would live, so what exactly was the problem? Besides, as an eleven-year-old, I would have been quite annoyed to wake up to pearly gates and not to my family.

As for my recovery, I set the record back in the day for the quickest recovery from such a surgery. I was possessed with a strange energy and excitement and restlessness. I put my all and more into my therapy and fitness and got out of the hospital in a mere four days.

We stayed in the hotel for about a month to be certain I was in the clear. During this time, I became addicted to hot showers for some reason. I took about four a day for around a year. This was also when I got my first and most obvious scar and deformity. It was not just an angry red scar, but a protrusion. I was never able to properly develop pecs as a result of it, the muscles cut and my ribcage broken in such a way that the scar always bulged forwards. It was far more sensitive back then, especially with the internal stitching still in there. It was like a long, extended paper clip stretched out under my skin. Touching it not only hurt, but reminded me of this metal visible below the surface. It has long since been removed, but I still occasionally get the sensation of steel beneath my skin there. Maybe I was a superhero from the surgery after all! However, even with this angry red thing, this weak spot, eventually I would have to go to school. It would be interesting to see how my classmates dealt with my recent changes. It would be interesting to see how I would deal as well.

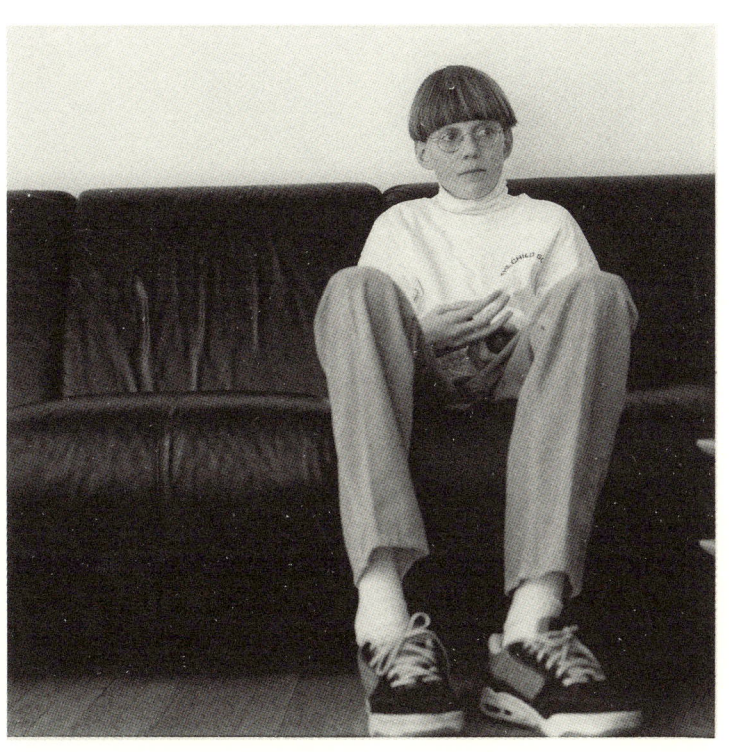

CHAPTER TWO:
A TALL GIRAFFE

There is a bit of a running joke at my old school. Do not worry; I will give you details on that in a moment, but I feel it is only right to start with this anecdote to set the stage.

    I was the biggest kid in class, always the biggest kid in class, without exception. At least in terms of height. I never had much in the way of muscle mass until much later in life after I stopped growing, as my bones expanded and lengthened far in advance of my lagging musculature. Therefore, I saw myself as a giraffe, one who is tall, used to being tall, not really caring for what he was born as, and thus neutral. I did not revile myself nor exalt myself for my condition: hence neutral.

    Now that I have explored the meaning of the title of the book, let us get back on track a bit. That being explaining that running joke I was talking of earlier, and to do that we'll need a small history lesson. I was big for a twelve-year-old when the fifth video game console generation (PlayStation, Nintendo 64, Sega Saturn) was just on its way out to make way for the sixth console generation (PlayStation 2, Nintendo GameCube, Sega Dreamcast, the original Xbox). Three-D Platformers and character action games, especially of the Collectathon and/or Mascot varieties, which were born in the fifth generation, rose to their heights in the sixth console generation; Jak and Daxter, Ratchet and Clank, Mario, Sonic. This was my world. Fascination and obsession took hold as my world became a bit internal and very challenging.

    One thing that is nearly ubiquitous to gaming is the *Boss Battle*. A confrontation with a computer-generated enemy far above the rank-and-file AI "enemies" that precede them, and thus their "Boss." Not always literally within the plot of the game, but often enough that the term stuck and became the jargon for all such enemies and challenges, my enemies, my challengers.

In addition, *Platformers* are defined as games that focus upon navigating complex series of obstacles (often some manner of floating platform, thus the genre) more so than complex combat mechanics. This results in Bosses that are big, intimidating, and which also have huge, often glowing weak spots that will kill them quickly when pummeled and jumped on enough times. The challenge becomes reaching their weak spots more so than fighting the Boss itself, often involving a lot of jumping from platform to platform.

And thus, the running gags at school. I was big, intimidating looking with a big, glowing weak spot in the form of my scar, and more importantly the weak heart underneath. The joke was that, for all my fearful size and stature, a few quick jabs at my scar would take me down with relative ease, just like in a video game.

I am certain now, as an adult, that a few jabs from my fellow elementary school peers would have failed to cause my heart to explode the way my friends and I thought back in those innocent days. Innocent days where the ebb and flow of your life could be measured on what game you were currently working through at the time and school assignments. But I am glad none of us were dumb enough to test the theory. While I could likely take most hits sent my way, I would always be rolling the dice. The chance of hitting snake eyes was always there. This was my first real encounter with my new physical limitations.

I cannot play contact sports, and really should avoid sports altogether, but the doctors left that up to my parents and me. While three mighty blows to my molten, glowing scar will most likely not take me down like some video game dragon, it did come from a place of truth. My elementary school chums did not come upon this joke by intuition. Someone told them, to the best of their ability, what my neat and ugly (with kids that young, those were correlated) new scar was all about.

That someone was me. I tried to convey to my friends what my doctors told me following my recovery. They told me of the moratorium on all contact sports, and I asked why. They told me that hard physical impacts to my chest, particularly the area around my scar, could lead to negative medical consequences—some potentially lethal. Of course, the eleven-year-old me latched onto that and exaggerated it in my head.

Therefore, I did indeed tell them, my classmates, that a fist to the chest could kill me. This spread to the rest of the school. There were two halves of my schools, something that I will go into detail later. Just know there were both high school and elementary students. I am fairly certain the high school kids were probably aware that things weren't quite that cut and dry, but the idea that you could kill the freakishly tall elementary school kid with one punch tickled their fancies, and as we all know teenagers are the worst. So they too spread the story as I told it. And thus, a legend was born in my school.

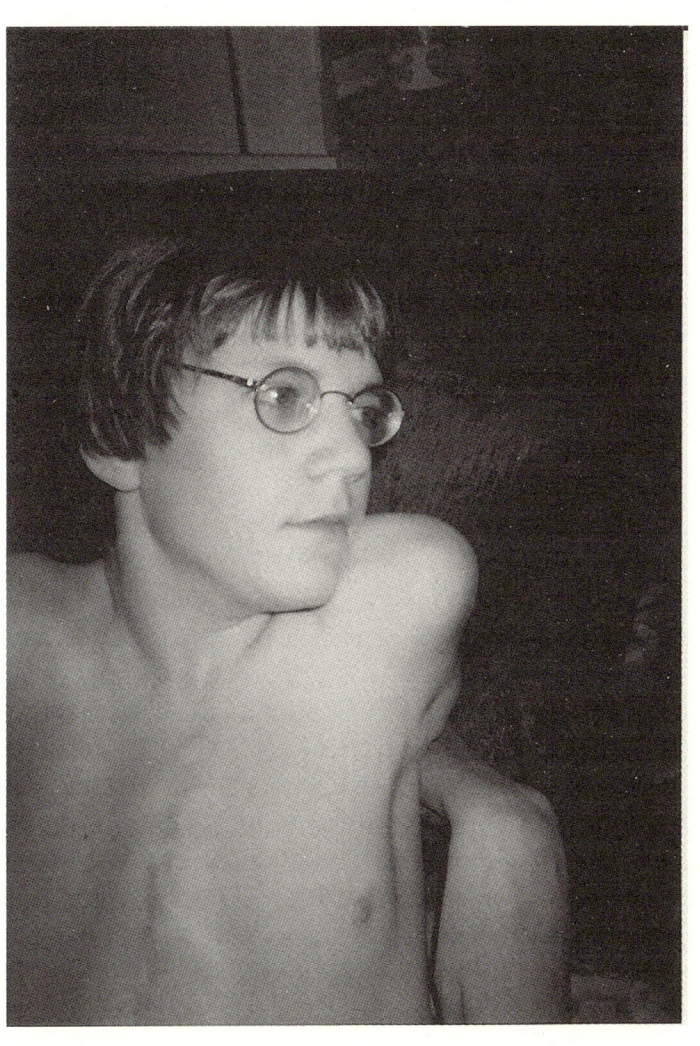

Upon reading all of that, there is a fair chance you are now expecting a large segment to be dedicated towards how I handled bullies in my life, to perhaps serve as warning or as an example for those with Marfan syndrome (be they readers or the readers' loved ones). While some may be sprinkled throughout the rest of the text, as I was not a complete stranger to bullying, I will have to apologize and say that there really won't be much in the way of this.

The reason for this is that... well, I was rarely bullied, something that would be outright unbelievable in hindsight for me (given what a weird child I was) if I did not also glean the full context behind this insulation. Insulation really is the right word here; because I avoided all this because others in some manner protected me from it. With my parents, it is the fact that they made sure I would never go to public school. While a lifetime of private education does come with some cons, particularly how much of a shock to the system university was, the fact that you can pick the right school certainly makes avoiding hostile environments for your child a lot easier. For my friends, as my friend Tommy shares, I was sort of the unwitting social glue holding our friend group back in New York City together and so this meant that they deliberately avoided getting me involved in any of the drama that would make these relationships rocky once I left. As I said, I was insulated.

This can be seen in how the times I was bullied severely; it never lasted long and only ever occurred when I left these insulated circles. I faced bullying when going on a cruise ship and attempted to make friends with the normal kids on board. I faced bullying at the playgrounds outside of school contexts. I faced it when I made myself noticeable at the arcade. I was insulated and had very little knowledge of what to do when I left that insulation.

Not that I ever needed to learn to deal back then. I was, at most, away from this safety net for about a few weeks. So, I weathered these bouts of confusing misery for a short time before my friends and family went back to protecting me. Thus, I am sorry to say that I am unfortunately not a wellspring of advice on what to do in cases of bullying.

I want to start at the beginning with The Child School. Depending on how one defines things, it was the first school I ever attended. I say "depends on how you define things" because I did, technically, attend a preschool before starting kindergarten at The Child School. But let us be honest with ourselves, preschools are glorified day care centers, and my parents were both very busy at this junction of my life. The Child School was where I began kindergarten and went on to attend elementary/grade school. Then came junior high, if we wish to use the more glamorous title, but let us call it middle school.

Let me discuss what I meant by "the other half" of the school. The Child School is not the full name of the institution, nor is Legacy High School a separate establishment, at least not entirely. The full name of the school is, quite the awkward one I might add, The Child School/Legacy High School. Not elegant by any means, and rather confusing, so let me explain. You see, the school was K-12, yet The Child School was not exactly the sort of name for a high school that any teen would be at all comfortable attending. The poor teenagers are already dealing with puberty, so humiliating them further with such a childish name for their institution was like rubbing salt in a wound. Thus, the school was effectively split into two names despite being one institution. The Child School took care of grade school; Legacy High School took care of the high school grades. Although middle school technically fell under The Child School name, there was so much staff overlap between the two programs that it was effectively a shared thing.

I remember joking to a classmate once that if the elementary school and high school represented both parts of The Child School/Legacy High School, then us middle school students, which we were when I concocted this quip, were represented by the and "/" or symbol.

This is my long way around to simply state that no matter what grade I was in, I shall henceforth only refer to this school as The Child School. This was because I was only ever tangentially involved with the Legacy High School half of the organization through my time in middle school. It was a private school (but a very affordable one; anyone could attend) that specialized in special education. The school covered physical disabilities and emotional and psychological ones, though for the most part it was the latter cases that drew in applicants. I was no exception. While my Marfan syndrome was certainly a factor in my parents deciding to keep me out of public education, I was enrolled into The Child School before my final Marfan diagnosis. I was about five and a half when I started kindergarten there, so it was about a year before I got my proper diagnosis.

My folks enrolled me at this institution for the next decade not due to my flawed heart, but rather my scrambled mind. I was diagnosed with severe ADHD and high functioning autism long before I got a confirmation on that tentative Marfan syndrome diagnosis from way back in Florida. This was all for the best as that was pretty much the specialty of Marie Desouza's life's work.

Marie was the owner, founder, and head administrator of The Child School/Legacy High School. While a private school devoted entirely to special education and serving the disabled is not exactly commonplace, it certainly was not unheard of or even uncommon. It was not an unheard-of thing when she was trying to get The Child School (TCS) off the ground. However, in many ways she broke ground, and paved the way for those who would come later.

Honestly, her life would make for the perfect Hollywood Oscar award-winning film. She was a true pioneer with noble goals in pushing boundaries, but also a flawed person. I remember a great number of strange moments in my life from school that were the result of severe overreaction and overcorrection on her part, bordering on the superstitious. For example, there was her absolute moratorium upon all things *Pokémon* related back to when the Pokémania of the 1990s and early 2000s were at their peak. We, by which I mean my fellow schoolmates and I, needed to use code language when trying to talk about the franchise, as even uttering the word Pokémon could land you in hot water. This was tough for many of us as we were gamers. As a school memory, it has many negative connotations.

I felt that I needed to establish that she was an eccentric to give context to much of what I am discussing. She and the school went above and beyond in so many ways, so I need you to understand that some of what I speak of is not mere flight of fancy or the creation of the ADHD mind. The "above and beyond" attitude extended to the severely negative aspects, so that should put aside any thought that this must be too good to be true, because it came at a price.

I started my academic career at the kindergarten level, age five-and-a-half. Unlike every other kid at that age, I never cared to keep track of the exact fraction of my age so I will say I was five. I also only recently had started to talk a few months earlier. I was very much a late bloomer in that regard, so much so that my parents feared that I would go through my life as a mute. Luckily, none of the other kids knew that, nor did I ever bring attention to it. Not because I was at all smart enough to keep it to myself to avoid bullying, but to be honest, at that age, really any age before my late teens, I did not think like that and would just blabber whatever embarrassing fact about me that came to mind. Rather, it did not even occur to me that it was anything of importance to begin with. It just did not come up.

Things were a tad different at this early juncture. I was always big for my age, but back then I was not so big as to be special in that regard. I was just a big kid then, not *The Tree*. That was my sometimes complimentary, sometimes insulting, depends on the speaker and the weather, nickname through most of my time at TCS. It was never maliciously used though. I had some bullies outside of school, but not in school. As I have said before, this baffled me for the longest time when I look back on those days, as even within this group of the strange and bizarre, I was an awkward child/teen. I recently came to realize that my best friend Tommy Fisher and I were the glue holding together many friend groups and cliques at TCS. This was more due to Tommy's conscious efforts and my own unconscious bumbling into people's lives than any plot of mine. This was evident in the fact that, once both Tommy and I left New York, things sure changed. Here is Tommy using his own special words and speech pattern:

> When I found out that our old friend group pretty much disintegrated when we both moved out of the state (New York), I admit that I was kind of shocked to learn that we were the social glue holding them together. I do mostly think that yes, kind of no but mostly yes, because

when we were around like most of our friends at school and I really like to describe it that we were unintentional ringleaders. It wasn't so much that we were trying to be like the boss of everybody. However, if something went wrong, one of us would be around to help the person out and you need that in a lot of social groups! You know everybody is different and I have opinions and they have opinions and somebody's gonna get mad. But when you left in 2005 and went to Arizona with your family, you know things were kind of still OK. You know we were friends, were still really close enough so we really missed you because we made it feel like it wasn't the same old crap in our classroom as we always said that you were the most eccentric one. You were so special in our eyes so when you left, it was kind of like everything started going from "let's do this, gamers" to "yeah, how's it chillin'?" We were close and everything. However, when older, that is when the politics started coming out. I do not mean just world politicians with that; I'm also talking like office politics. There was the competition between homerooms. Without you to just ignore that and obliviously force everyone back together because you didn't care, everything started breaking down. You were the glue. (Tommy Fisher)

This means in retrospect that I was in fact above being bullied beyond a good-natured ribbing over what a weird *Tree* I was. That nickname was bestowed because I was tall and skinny, thus a tree. Trust me, I am no mountain of a man after all, and even a Redwood looks thin when seen from a far. In many ways, I was very lucky at the school.

The school building that I attended for the elementary segment of my school career was this picturesque London type building in downtown New York City. Yes, that means I was in spitting distance of all those huge skyscrapers. I was right there for 9/11. I can tell you I remember that day quite vividly. Maybe it was because I remember the smell of all the backed-up cars. Interesting that my other issues do not allow me to have such vivid memories, but this one is still fresh in my mind. Maybe it is because New York City and all its buildings were my home. Or perhaps it is something a bit more obvious, that on that day history was made and for the absolute worse.

Such was the case with my old venerable schoolhouse that looked like a building you would find in London and not New York City, though it admittedly had to contend with far more monolithic neighbors. I remember it as well. It was also very small, and the fact that it was able to semi-comfortably fit hundreds of students from kindergarten to middle school and on to surly high school kids is quite frankly miraculous. It helped that it had an oversized basement.

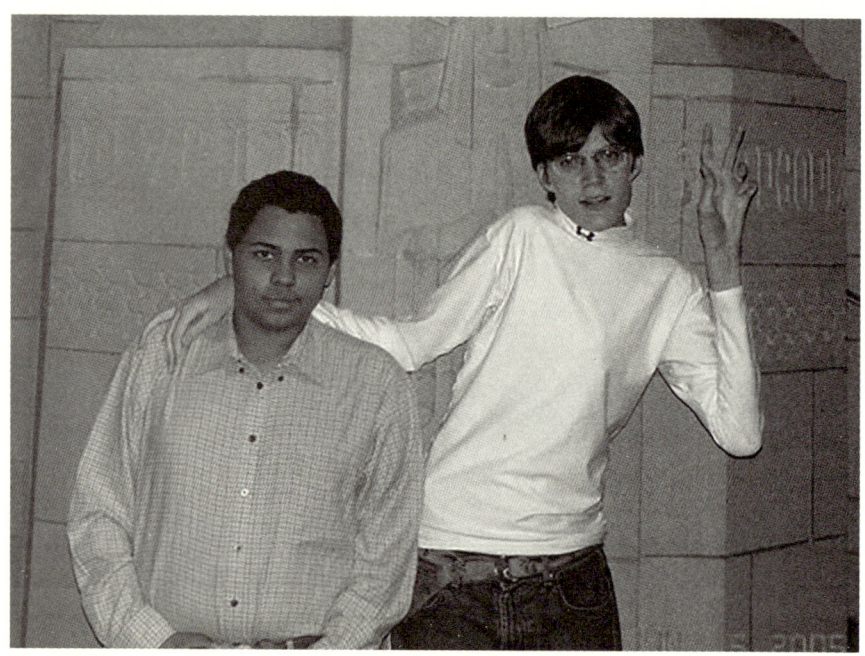

At age 12, I was already showing signs of severe scoliosis that would dangerously start to shift my heart from my left side to my right.

Eventually, the gentlemanly old building was going to reach its limits as hundreds of more parents sought the best for their disabled children and thus the whole "Raise the Roof" initiative began. The plan was to add five new stories on top of what was formerly our roof. We got about one new story before it became prohibitively expensive. Ultimately, despite all the t-shirts and other merchandise that the school had produced to celebrate and help fund this event, despite all the hype and all my classmates and I thinking of progressively grander and grander ideas for these new floors, nothing truly came of it. I do admit that my creative mind thought of many ways to raise money! Instead, when I was thirteen and starting middle school, the administration sold the building and moved to Roosevelt Island, New York.

To me, Roosevelt Island was a strange place, frankly in some ways like another planet altogether to this New York City boy. Obviously, almost none of us lived there, but the new school was indeed there to stay. It was a permanent occupation of territory, a permanent outpost and base if you would, perhaps even a colony, one under the flag of us out-of-towners. I think we were invaders!

This time, the invaders did indeed intend to stay. To say this caused some sparks to fly would certainly not be a lie. There were quite a few confrontations between the older school kids and the locals: turf wars. I should clarify that I am talking about the local kids here. We got a few glares and some sour attitudes from the adults, but they gave my classmates and me no trouble beyond that. I do know there was some friction between the teachers/school administration and the local shop owners, but I was never privy to any of that. I only ever came to know of these turf wars by conversations after the fact with those who were involved. My memory was not the best for these things.

Well, that is not entirely true. I remember some bruised high school kids and glares from across the street, and suddenly finding myself with what I now know looking back to be an honor guard of sorts when locals got close. It seems that my reputation for fragility, due to my Marfan syndrome, had made it so that I was deliberately kept as far from the worst of it as possible. They did not go out of the way to keep me in the dark though; it is just that back then I was an incredibly oblivious kid, head always in the clouds. Marfan syndrome gave me other problems at other times as well.

To give an example, when I was about nine, I had to deal with a particularly rude metro driver (the local public buses). He seemed intent on denying me entry to the bus, even though at that age I was entitled to get on free and without question. I was eventually let on, and I forgot all about the rude man as he ultimately did his job, and I was too focused on training my *Pokémon*.

However, there was a bit more going on there than just some random jerk abusing his power. As you likely know by now, either dealing with the condition yourself or of a loved one, Marfan syndrome causes one to grow abnormally fast. Nobody seems to know exactly why this is the case, though due to the condition being possibly genetic some assume that the genes for bone growth might be related somehow. Thus, the reason for the driver's initial denial was because he thought I was some smug teenager trying to get on the bus for free by posing as a nine-year-old. I was that tall. This was very awkward for everyone. It took my babysitter pulling out my birth certificate to get me on, but again, I was quite oblivious to all this until much later in life. I took so much in stride.

Getting back to TCS, I was no different than other kids—we had field trips, and they were amazing. First, we had the spring trips! These were particularly ostentatious. This was a real above and beyond moment for our school. I say this because all such trips were out of the country or, at the very least, out of the mainland in the case of American territories out in the Pacific and in the Caribbean. We did occasionally go to places within the mainland, such as Boston and D.C., but that was the exception.

To say this was unusual would be putting it mildly, but because I was an oblivious kid and this is all I have ever known, I thought that all schools regularly toured Central America and went island hopping. Honestly, they really should. I may have become somewhat jaded to Eurasia as of late, but I maintain that Americans really should become as familiar with our own backyard as Europeans are with theirs. It is fun, as I recall.

There was one year we went to Europe, but for the most part the trips were confined to the Americas. But still, there was a huge list of potential destinations within such criterion.

It was through these spring trips that I discovered my love for Costa Rican coffee. We got it straight from the source. Columbian coffee can shove off my friends! I enjoyed the travel more than I can say.

There was one time in the Bahamas when my condition, the one this book is about, came into play. I got a nasty cut on my foot. Calling it a cut is not entirely accurate. A loose piece of broken off pool flooring bored an almost perfectly circular hole in the sole of my foot. It spilled enough blood to not look out of place in a *Jaws* film. That part of the pool started to look like Hawaiian Punch, is what I am saying. This happened during a dunking war.

What is a *dunk war* you ask? Why, that is when all the elementary and middle school students unite to swarm the gym teachers and the high school kids try to dunk them into the pool, and I do mean swarm. The gym teacher had five kids crawling over him trying to force him into the pool at any one time; he then flung them off into the water. The gym teacher was the goal of all this. He had an honor guard of high school students and everything. Yes, not the sort of thing my doctors would approve of me being involved in, but at the time that sort of thing barely crossed my mind. Well, I got that hole in my foot from all of that. It quickly reminded me I had Marfan.

It would be a concern of the teachers if this happened to any of their charges, but worse for me with Marfan syndrome. They quite rightly overreacted. They had no idea how this would interact with my ailment, so instead of just getting a cast, I was made wheelchair bound for the rest of the trip. What a great reminder that I was different—not.

You are all probably thinking this trip all cost an arm and a leg, and while it certainly wasn't cheap, it was surprisingly affordable. It was just $400 per student. Marie was good at finding deals for these sorts of things. It was one of the plusses that she gave to the school.

Now onto the other big thing that the school did that was above and beyond the call of duty: the June plays.

These plays might as well have been professional, with all the effort we put into them. Seriously, I'm pretty sure we could have taken them on the road and made a tidy little profit. And unlike the spring trips, parents did not have to pay a dime for this. Though there were in fact a lot of June play donation drives leading up to the performance, these were purely voluntary. We just did not need the money.

In addition, the productions we decided to take on were not the usual sterilized versions of Shakespeare and Arthurian Mythology you are likely conjuring in your heads. No, frankly we did a lot of too much adult stuff. We did *The Producers* and *Rocky Horror Picture Show*. I played the gay director in the former and the criminologist in the latter. I guess I want you all to see that I was not limited in what I did at my school by Marfan. In fact, I do not think I gave it a second thought at the time. I just joined in.

In fact, I loved it all, though looking back, I have absolutely zero clue how the school got away with the many things they did. What you may have noticed in all of this, beyond some weird jokes and urban legends started by my friends and school acquaintances, is how little my having Marfan syndrome comes up. That is because, at this point in my life, my condition did not really affect me directly outside of a few isolated occurrences here and there. And almost all of these involved how it caused others to perceive me as opposed to how the condition affected me. I never really knew how I was being perceived by fellow classmates with Marfan until Tommy let me know:

> You were, and I hope this doesn't sound too bad, you were a spectacle at the school because here you are TALL and oh how I remember to this day when a kid named Dylan Hamilton tried to make a stick as tall as you. Yeah, I remember that and I think people really are neat you know. They kinda really cared about you and in some way shape or form

even if they're not your friend per se because you, and all puns intended here, you really **STOOD** out in the school. Do you know what I mean? They don't see some freak with Marfan, it's just that all they see is a really tall white kid. (Tommy Fisher)

There it is, the running joke about my glowing weak point, being *The Tree* that I started this chapter with, and the anecdote about the bus driver misjudging my age for access. It was all about how I was perceived, not who I really was. However, this all began to change as I entered my late teens and moved to Arizona.

CHAPTER THREE:
ARIZONA BOUND

I am hoping that by now you may have noticed what my coping mechanism has been for my Marfan syndrome. My coping mechanism is not to cope at all. Yes, it is all just normal here in *Christopia*. There is no chronic pain where I live. You will see that this will continue a little longer, and in many ways, it continues even to this day in some format. It is just that I am far more conscious of it in the present.

Again, it is why I chose the title of my story that I did! To me, a giraffe really does not care that it is not a water buffalo or anything grandiose, nor does it think of itself some freakish mutant horse. No, it is just what it is: a giraffe. It does not exalt in being a giraffe, nor does it envy the horse or hold it in any ill will. It simply is. Of course, in later years, when this giraffe gets hit right in the face with a billion and one exclusive ailments all at once in a very short period, then he starts to envy those dang water buffalo.

What will eventually come to an end is my ability to just flatly ignore my Marfan syndrome. For the longest time, the first sixteen or so years of my life to give a more exact number, Marfan syndrome barely existed. It was the thing that sent me to the doctor's office and was the source of "hit his weak point for massive damage" jokes in my childhood. It was also the reason I was not supposed to exercise as much as most kids (which suited me just fine back then, sedentary nerd that I was). I never just flat out forgot that I had it, but outside those rare occasions listed, it really did not exist. Not even my height kept it in focus. True, Marfan syndrome is the source of that for me, but not all tall people (even ridiculously tall folks) have the condition. After all, the modern NBA simply would not work if all their star players were at risk with every chest impact. I was in the "coping by not coping" stage until we moved to Arizona!

I was about fifteen at the time. It should be noted that, at least in this instance, this move was not prompted in any way by my medical conditions. Nope, they were prompted by my Mom's.

At the time, she was suffering with crippling degrees of stress. Yeah, Mom had pretty much reached her last rope, and she needed to retire. While it will end up being semi-retirement (at best) in reality, it was why we moved. Mom retired from show biz! Perhaps I should go into at least a bit of detail on this point. You see, Mom was a very busy woman. Dad, in this case Peter (and boy do I hate having to constantly make that distinction; both Peter and Jim have earned that moniker in my eyes, and when I'm with one or the other, I simply refer to them as Dad) was also a fairly busy man. However, Peter was freelance, a freelance sportswriter to be exact, so while he often went to an office to do his literary work, he just as often wrote from home. Thus, he was rarely gone. However, Mom was a different case entirely.

Unlike Dad, she often found herself flung from one end of the country to the other, and that was when she was not being flung from one end of the world to the other. Florida, Britain, and France were a few of the frequent locations that her profession dragged her to. But truly, I do not believe there is a state in our nation she has not stepped foot in. She has been from one end of Eurasia to another as well. Wherever she was summoned, she went. It was her professional obligation and her life, and it was taking a toll on her well-being. Something had to change, and I guess for them, Arizona was the answer.

I honestly think I would have gone through at least high school before we moved elsewhere if Mom and Dad had different professions. Dad has quite happily settled into retirement now and was content enough to be something of a house husband at the time (not really one obviously, just being my flippant self). I also feel Dad probably had more of a stomach for what mom went through than she did.

Mom was a dyed-in-the-wool, globetrotting dancer for a good chunk of her life, but by the time she had me, she had something of an obsession with her son, and rightly so. I do not believe leaving my side as frequently as she did was something she much desired, and she would have loved being able to work from home. Mom was not the sort that could be content by just keeping house. But writing from home like Dad, with myself a mere few rooms away, would have made her very happy.

The sort of company she had to keep due to her profession was also not helping; this was show business. This was my mom, Ann Reinking, and well, she had to do her thing for the family, especially me. I think she was worried about finances in the beginning:

OK for myself, I had some investments that have dividends coming in and I also continued to teach dance and choreograph and then I had an opportunity to choreograph the show *Chicago*. I also got to be in it for a certain amount of time, as the main character, and that became a big hit on Broadway and that was a big break for all of us! But at first, I didn't have money of my own and I had been living off investments/living off of dividends, but it really helped you know. That changed when *Chicago* became a success. I always have money coming in from working because of that. I started working a time choreographing and teaching dance at University. But when you were little, I had to supplement my investments with working. Plus, I was told by your teachers at the *Child Development Center*, as well as my own therapist, to work because I needed to be happy and to feel like I was doing something proactive for you as well as for me. I needed to know that there was money coming in because I did worry about money in the beginning and then later and happy *Chicago* took off. (Ann Reinking)

There is a joke in my house that is still told that was connected to my Mom's destined retirement. Mom, the initial origin of the joke, was having anger issues that were akin to a nuclear weapon. It was a huge explosion with radiation that left the house deadly to all life forms for days to come. Mom had been deploying her nuclear arsenal more and more frequently in the last days in New York. That was it. It was time for her to retire and move out of the stressful city to the nation's retirement capital: Phoenix, Arizona.

I would specify the suburbs, but that would imply anybody actually lived in the city. No, people work in the city, and that is it. I soon learned that the "City" was nothing like my beloved New York City. I do remember my first day in Arizona. By that, I mean my first day off the plane after we moved to Arizona. We had, of course, flown out several times to check out what the heck we were getting ourselves into, but that first day was memorable.

I remember going into the airport garage and thinking, "Oh my God, we moved out of the city into a literal oven!" Seriously, I could see the heat rising from the ground and wafting off the walls!

This experience was all due to ignorant city folk mentality. If our present day selves were to hop in a time traveling Delorean to tell our past selves anything... well, first I'd tell past me to just jump into writing instead of getting trapped in University for a decade due to medical concerns before anything else, but secondly, I'd tell him and my folks to not move to Phoenix during the summer! I am pretty sure we moved to Arizona in August! This was indeed the first of many adjustments.

We did not immediately move into what would be my home for the next eight years and still my parents' home to this day. We stayed in a house rental for about four months while we waited for that place to become ready for habitation. The rental place was nice, beyond nice. The place we eventually moved into is, by most objective standards, so much better. However, I greatly preferred the rental. I have never mentioned this to my parents so upon reading this book, they will now be aware of my bias in living accommodations. After all, my "room" was a smaller mini house! It was great! It was on the other side of the pool from the main house. I felt autonomous.

I am not going to go into any greater detail on the place. One is because it is frankly irrelevant to my various ailments or towards my greater life story. It was a transitory place, after all, a way station. Also, because my memories of the place are quite fuzzy, but that is pretty much the story of my life. After all, it was a short stop in my life; how many gas stations do you recall?

I will share a final detail though. I watched the absolute hell out of a collector's DVD box set of the *Star Wars Original Trilogy*, long before the public began to forgive and reevaluate the quality of the Prequels, and long before the Sequel Trilogy was even a dream of Bob Iger's. This box set even came with the documentary, *Empire of Dreams*, detailing Lucas's early career and the creation of the *Original Trilogy*. Brilliant stuff that you should all check out when you have the chance!

I watched those three films (that being the actual *Star Wars* films) a lot. I also watched the documentary quite frequently, but not to the literal autistic level I watched the actual science fiction classics, which was quite literally hundreds of times. I cannot give an actual number because I lost count. Seriously, why would I keep count? I was a teen enjoying his favorite films! Besides, you remember me, the one with the faulty memory for numbers. How am I so certain I watched them literally hundreds of times then? It was because I became so familiar with the films that I could quote the trilogies script back-to-back. It was like karaoke, but with film scripts. Come to think of it, maybe it was part of my autism. However, I still impressed the hell out of my parents. Sadly, the fun had to end and, during this time at the rental, we started to go school hunting.

Not much noticeably happened during this time that I care to share. Eventually, we found Gateway Academy, my next high school. I would go into a lot of detail on this one but let us say there is a lot of personal baggage here and leave it at that. Some details will come to light later, as this is where I graduated from high school, so it is inevitable, but nothing beyond that which is strictly necessary. This was a school for those on the autism spectrum, and I do feel that they were ill equipped to handle my Marfan syndrome. There were high spots and low spots at school. I missed my best friend Tommy and feel that I was ripped away not only from the only lifestyle I had ever known and had become comfortable with, but also from my closest school chum. It was traumatic on one hand and adventurous on the other. Such is autism. I think Tommy really sums up what being friends is like while having autism:

> Well, you know me! As a kid, I never was very judgmental of anybody, but first thing I thought was, "he was much taller than most of the other kids" and boy did we laugh. But as you know they say autistic people know each other much better than other people, we couldn't actually talk but somehow do you know it's kind of how you are. There's something about autistic people that even when we are talking and we're having a good conversation, there's something about the way we talk, the way we look at each other, the way we present to each other that even when we're older I noticed and you go "Oh shoot, we were the same! She's like me or he's like me!" You know what I'm saying? (Tommy Fisher)

Yes Tommy, I know exactly what you are saying, as neither one of us could say at what age we met with accuracy. Also, what the nature of the relationship is. However, I do miss those good times and was hoping that my new school would bring new friendships as I kept the old ones dear to my heart. I also knew I had to do more than just academics and the hunt was now on for a physical therapist. For you see, in all this, I was still medically required, thanks to Marfan, to seek out physical therapy.

We found ourselves a physical therapist by the name of John Greer. He is no longer my therapist as such, but he is still one of my best friends and we still work out together, but in a far more specialized manner. He was a three-time world champion in Tae Kwon Do. Through him, I learned I had both a talent and passion for the martial arts; finally, a controlled contact sport. I was having a great time. I was on top of the world in my own little world. It is obvious even to me now, that I was still in that coping without coping mode. However, my armor was about to crack. Will *Christopia* start to crumble?

CHAPTER FOUR:
LIMITATIONS

Wow! The end of Chapter Three was a bit of a cliffhanger. Maybe it is because my life at that point seemed like one; maybe, life imitating art? I seem to gravitate towards viewing my life through the filter of literary conventions. Honestly, that is just how I tend to view reality, through the filter of fiction. However, this "literary filter" does work into my coping mechanisms.

It looks like I have been ripping through my life story at a rapid pace. That is because while I am telling my life story, I am telling it as it pertains to coping with Marfan syndrome. Well that, and because I decided that a brisk pace makes for the best read for this sort of material. Let us be fair with ourselves, most of our lives are made of some fairly dry, uninteresting stuff. For the first sixteen years of my life, it was easy to ignore I even had Marfan. Now, the condition became something I had to directly contend with, and not simply a passive burden. It is time to finally start delving into those details of the next four years of my life. I shall begin with John Greer.

I am certain the giraffe wanted to protect himself from the lions and wanted to look good doing it. He went out to find someone to teach him. He found this teacher, in a meercat of all things. A lifelong friendship was formed that day. Now with this fairly ham-fisted crack at John's height and attempt to tie it back to the title out of the way, let us get back to it.

I finally found a physical sport I was both good at and was passionate about. It is unfortunate that said sport was not only a contact sport, but a combat sport on top of that. However, it led me to meet a wonderful gentleman that I can sincerely call friend. As mentioned, I require regular physical therapy. Well, I did at the time. I am uncertain how needed it is now. I used to need a thousand and one therapists to attend to me. Now, I have a psychiatrist and a physical therapist, and frankly the therapist feels more like a basic physical trainer who any Dick or Jan would employ to stay fit, or at least put on the appearance of maintaining fitness. However, when I first met John, I still needed my thousand and one therapists.

What this all comes down to is that, when we found John, we were not looking for someone qualified as an instructor in the martial arts. We were looking for a physical therapist to help with managing my Marfan syndrome as it pertained to my physical fitness. We initially hired John on his merits (of which there are many) in physical fitness and his medical knowledge. He is also quite accomplished in the latter because he is a former Marine medic.

John's life story is quite fascinating, enough so that I have written several characters based upon said life for other (unpublished at the time of this writing) works of mine. However, I will give a very brief rundown here, just so everyone knows where he is coming from. John was born in Hawaii and is of Scottish descent. He was one of the few white kids in his school, which made him a target of bullying and worse. Short and narrow of it, he got beaten up a lot over this. Combine this with some home life issues and a healthy diet of Bruce Lee, John became interested in the martial arts to defend himself. With proper training and his stint in the military as a medic, he became a great candidate to be my new physical therapist!

The best part is that when he eventually re-entered civilian life, he fully devoted himself to the martial arts and fitness as a career, particularly Tae Kwon Do with the ATA (American Tae Kwon Do Association). He went on to become the ATA World Champion three times. He then got accredited as both a licensed physical therapist and a teacher for the ATA. This sealed the deal for me (and a bit more importantly, my parents).

Since my parents already secured a school, they then found and hired John. By this point, we had been living in Arizona somewhere between half a year and a full year. I was still very new to the state, but I was settled in by that point and now completely understood this was not a vacation. I was now well accustomed to the idea that I was here to stay, even if I did not really think of the place as my home. Personally, I still do not really see the state of Arizona as my home. When I am away, I never miss the desert and suburbia itself the way I missed New York City when returning from being away for any length of time. But here I am and here I will remain for now, at least.

I was happy that my parents liked John. They certainly were not looking for martial arts instruction. While there was a lot of overlap between his martial arts students and his physical therapy clients (I was an example of such), he had plenty of people he saw in only one capacity or the other. Honestly, at the time, I am pretty sure my parents would have balked at my practicing martial arts, with all the physical contact and such.

My parents hired him on as my physical therapist. He did train me at my place when needed, but usually I went to his gym. Much of what he needed to do with me required workout machines my family did not own. For a while that was what John was to me: my physical therapist, there to help me manage the fitness side of having Marfan syndrome but whom I knew instructed others in martial arts.

As I mentioned earlier, I was very much the sedentary nerd type as far as interests were concerned. Not truly "sit down all day in front of a television/computer, every day, without exception" type, as I had way too much nervous energy. However, I was not the type to relish exercising beyond the bare minimum. While I found John's Tae Kwon Do routines to be fascinating to observe, I had for a time little desire to add that on top of the workout routine that John was already having me do. This did not last long, just a few months in fact. I am uncertain what exactly changed my mind, though I do know it was something of a buildup. A lot of things pushed me to ultimately ask him to train me. Partly it was because I wondered what he thought about me. I asked John what his thoughts were when he first met and started to work with me:

> I remember that day well. Both your father and mother were present and introduced us. Despite the usually high fitness traffic and energetic vibe at Pure Fitness, you were very outgoing and polite. Initially, was a little concerned, given your progressively deforming frame at the time, due to the Marfan syndrome. With your awesome attitude, for the most part, your participation and progressions in balance and coordination soon put any concerns I initially had to rest. (John Greer)

The point here is that I literally had years of pop culture, and my own intense fascination and curiosity pressuring me to ask John to teach me martial arts. I think I was normal in this more than I knew at the time. I grew up with films and cartoons and anime about martial artists and, most importantly here, students learning from Masters.

Hear me out—Daniel learning from Mister Miyagi and overcoming Cobra Kai in *The Karate Kid* Films, Jackie Chan learning from Uncle (and Jade likewise learning from Jackie in the cartoon *Jackie Chan Adventures*. Yes, that was a thing that existed and was a far better show than it had any right to be. On that subject add Jackie Chan films like *Rush Hour* and *Shanghai Knights*. Goku and God knows how many instructors he had over the course of the *Dragon Ball* shows, becoming a planet destroying Godling through dedication to Kung Fu alone—and I do mean planet destroying; a legitimate concern in later parts of the show was to make sure special attacks only graze the ground and not directly hit it as to avoid detonating the planet. I was sixteen, so Naruto and his quest to become the Hokage, as well as his many mentors like Kakashi and Jiraiya, would also be an influence. Yes, he may have been a ninja and not strictly a martial artist, but that is splitting hairs. On that subject, let us include Splinter and the Ninja Turtles. You can say I was quite influenced!

While I may not remember exactly what triggered me to go and ask John, I am pretty sure I know the general process that led me to that decision. Amazing how I can remember process more than actual events or decisions. I figured I would give it a try, see if it is for me. Hopefully, I would not completely suck at this. How would I ever face my anime heroes if I did! Also, who knows, I jokingly considered if maybe John could teach me to channel my chi to summon beams of spiritual energy with megatons worth of destructive power, or how to cut through steel with a katana. The reality is why John would even want to work with me on this:

> In the world of martial arts, it is incumbent upon the instructor to provide each student with the challenges for personal growth on the path to black belt. If the student accepts, and with the instructor's guidance, forges the tenacity to accept these challenges thru learned tenacity, perseverance, and focus, the student will always find success in life as well as their "pil sung" on their path to black belt. While it's true both the Marfan and Asperger issues left us with unique challenges in your martial arts training, you met every challenge head on and never gave up. You persevered and as such discovered in yourself your ability to overcome many challenges. These abilities extended beyond merely your forms and weapon training. You also showed improvements at home and in school as well. (John Greer)

The fact that I learned to do something so spectacular in my eyes, even if only in theory, shows that this decision went a lot further than I could ever imagine. When I signed on, I would have been happy with learning to punch somewhat decently. Again, I expected to be either a complete screw up or just competent enough to muddle by. I did not expect to become John's star pupil and an actual legend in the ATA.

By actual legend, I mean a lot of folks doubted I even existed. Like, where did John find this wonder kid and why do we never see him at any tournaments? Yet the paperwork always passed muster. Either John Greer was some master forger the likes of which belongs in a Hollywood film, or else I did indeed exist. In the shadows, awaiting to emerge from the primordial fog, I was born to devour lesser students before once more ascending to the heavens with the Celestial Emperor. There goes that fiction writer in me, and this helps more than you know. Seems like *Christopia* was growing and not crumbling thanks to marital arts!

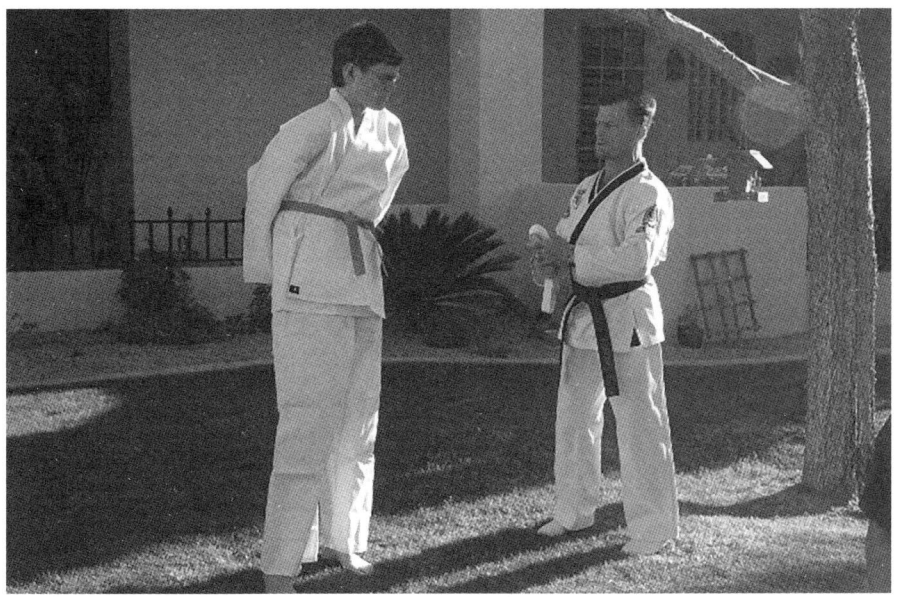

*John Greer presenting me with
my white belt in Tae Kwon Do*

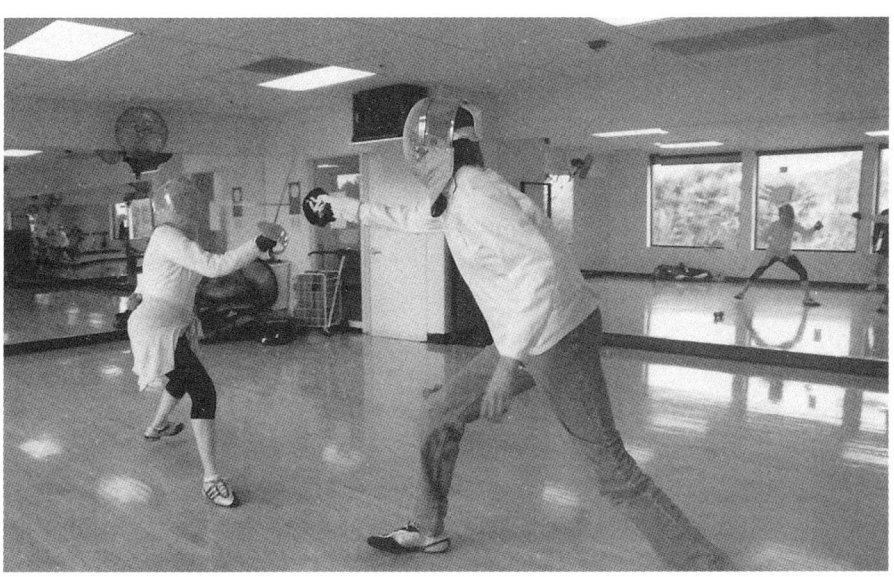

Fencing with Mom

Sadly, the reason I did not attend any tournaments, the reason I was some ghost, was something far more mundane and frankly tragic. The reason is because Marfan syndrome finally decided to directly interfere in my life. I found something I was good at, truly good at! It just so happened to be, in its competitive form, a combat sport. There was no way my doctors would ever approve of this. How was I going to justify this in my mind?

There were other options: form competitions and tournaments, to be precise. I was simply not interested in pursuing these though. Maybe I should have, but it really felt like a consolation prize. Sorry, we cannot let you into the real thing due to your minefield of a heart; have this instead. Unfair to those who put their all into those competitions, but that is how I felt. I initially rose through the ranks at a meteoric rate, blasting through most of the color belts in a few years. I only just finished learning my Black Belt form this year, and I am now thirty. I just want to remind you that I started doing this at age sixteen. This was the beginning of a long line of frustrations caused by the condition I once so easily ignored. I could not ignore it any longer. This is where the limitations came in.

I feel as though I should clarify some things here. You may be getting the impression that, based upon my testimony, Marfan syndrome only affects athletics and physical activity insofar as heavy contact is concerned. That is not the case. Special emphasis should be placed upon "I could ignore it no longer." The condition affects the heart, which is essential to physical activity and of course, as a consequence, athletics. Marfan syndrome will always have a direct effect upon sports and other athletic heavy activities (fun fact: boxing is technically not a sport due to the need for judges). I get winded faster than most, and I must regularly check my heart rate to make sure I do not go over a certain BPM (beats per minute). This severely limits the range of exercise one can engage in. Even at the height of my fitness, and I indeed got fit, I only had what could be called a swimmer's build. Yes, we folks with Marfan syndrome are likely never going to break into heavyweight boxing or bodybuilding levels of buff, which is a bit ironic considering how tall we get. Can you imagine a buff giraffe? Yes, Marfan syndrome always affected me in the realm of athletics and physical exercise, but I very easily adapted to and accepted those limitations. I simply did not care about those limitations the way I cared about the inability to fully engage in the martial arts.

I feel that a point of contrast on this situation would be the way none of this really bothered me at all during my fencing career, and it was technically a career. I was connected to the professional circuit. I trained under a man named Jim Barber, learning the ways of the saber. Now, one could not be faulted in thinking that fencing would count as contact, but apparently not. After years of competition, I can understand why. Even the hardest impacts barely bruise, and lightning quick taps were the optimal strategy, just light enough of a tap to complete an electrical circuit in your opponent's suit or mask as to have it register on the score sensor. Any attack with enough force to hurt is a dumb play, as such a move is so telegraphed within the context of fencing, that being quite fast, that even the freshest novice could block it with ease. I competed semi-professionally, as in I competed in professional circuit tournaments with prize pools without any expectation of going the whole way. I think I made something like $400 over the course of a decade of competing, and I did not care. Mom also competed alongside me, and she did better. That I was competing is the point.

Point is, I got good enough to qualify for these tournaments, but I never excelled at it. I think the biggest difference between fencing and martial arts is that the sport of martial arts is about self-mastery, instinct, and, most importantly for me, pattern recognition. Fencing on the other hand is often quite counter-intuitive as far as combat instincts are concerned and is essentially a physical chess match played at supersonic speeds with sabers instead of pieces. I am not good at chess. Thinking five moves ahead of my opponent is not my strong suit, so do not ask me to do that while said opponent is moving at apparent speeds that would not seem out of place in a superhero film. The biggest point here was that during the course of my less than successful semi-professional fencing career, at no point did my Marfan syndrome become apparent to me outside of being told to occasionally check my pulse and have frequent breaks.

Yet even here, where Marfan was finally affecting me directly and could not be ignored, this was only one area of my life.

Outside of my budding sports career, the status quo held. At least mostly. The high school I ended up attending was another private one, like last time. It was called Gateway Academy, and it focused specifically upon education for students with autism, as opposed to disabilities in general, which was the case of The Child School/Legacy High School in New York. I did not enter what one could call mainstream education until I started college, and I admit suddenly having to deal with peers whom, on average, did not have some measure of seen disability was something of a shock.

I cannot help but think I may have been better off gaining some experience with the mainstream population before suddenly being dumped into the ocean of the nominally normal and being told to swim. Perhaps my parents should have considered public school for me.

At Gateway, the fact that it was so focused upon autism meant I stood out quite a bit more by comparison to my time in TCS in New York City. I may have been the tallest elementary student (then junior high student), as well as the only one with Marfan syndrome in the student body. I was, however, by no means the only one with some manner of physical disability, and there were a few seniors who were taller than me. Anyone who knows how tall I ultimately got may find this a touch strange; let us just say that my current near seven-foot stature is somewhat artificial thanks to an impending surgery at the time. The point is that while I did stand out somewhat back then, I stood out a lot more in Gateway than I ever did back in the city. I never really knew the kind of first impression I made at the school. However, I did interview a few of the students for this writing and I found their views interesting. I am still friends with Robert, and it was good to hear this:

> When we first met, I thought you were the coolest freak of nature I had ever seen. Up until that point in my life, I viewed those with disabilities as people I could never get along with because I never understood them and felt I never could. With your personality, it was the first time I could see past the disability in front of me and see a person instead. (Robert)

I was still once more a freak in a school of freaks who knew they were freaks. I say that last bit with all affection possible by the way. I was a bit freakier than them, but not by such a degree that it was ever an issue. It was simply more obvious. They were in no position to get superior with me, at least in that regard, and they knew it. I wonder if this was a good thing. I mean, not getting bullied by them certainly was not a bad thing. While I may joke with my friends about how some particularly obnoxious members of the Millennial generation and Generation Z needed to be bullied more as kids, I never actually mean it, and I sure hope my friends didn't mean it either. Still, sometimes I really feel like I missed something, completely dodging the usual social jungle most teenagers must navigate. It was not as if my time in Gateway was completely devoid of all teasing and ribbing, but in the end, we were all friends there. Some of them I rightly should have not been friends with, and likely would have avoided if I were in a normal school environment, but it was frankly hard to avoid getting sucked into the clique when there were only about thirty other students attending Gateway. Frankly, I think I needed some rude awakenings: a few proverbial slaps to the back of the head, which I have only started receiving now with my current group of friends. I carried on a ton of bad habits through college that I feel I should have been weaned off of in high school, but wasn't because the student body was too small to afford much in the way of otherwise healthy conflict and competitiveness.

Who knew that some of the students also thought quite well of me, like Julie, one of the few girls at the school. "When I first met Chris, I thought he was a cool kid. I wondered why he was so tall and what the thing on his chest was. He seemed to be smart!" (Julie)

Gateway was also tiny. The Child School/Legacy High School was a small school. Only about 300 or so students, below average. Gateway was smaller, and at its absolute peak, had about 50 students. When I was there, it only had about 30 students or so. So that may have also contributed towards my bad self never becoming a target; everyone in the school essentially became one clique. Now that is something to think about unto itself, the entire school as a clique of well, a nice bunch of misfits. To be honest, I think we all enabled each other just enough to get by.

The teachers had a lot to deal with, especially with someone like me who fit in kind of. One of my teachers throughout my Gateway experience was Patricia Tusay.

She was a special education teacher who was certified in ASD but also taught at University. Honestly, I thought she was more of a pushover than most, but I soon found out she just really liked each one of us:

> I joined the school one term after it opened. I never really saw myself as a K-12 teacher, but having had my own issues in school, I wanted to work with all students not just college. Chris was different when I met him. I did not see him as being intellectually impaired in any way. He had physical limitations, but many of the students had sensory issues, so I called it an even match. He was above most of the students intellectually, in wit and common sense and it was great fun having him in the class as he set up a challenge for the others. I was new to Marfan and, when he first was at the school, he seemed limitless in what he could do to a large degree academically. We teachers planned lessons around Chris as to keep him engaged and to challenge the others as well. He was an incredible asset to the school. He kept us hopping! (Patricia Tusay)

So how did I manage to be just the giraffe that I always was? How I was uncaring and neutral as to my condition, in the jungle like social insanity that often defines high school? The truth is, I did not. I never had to deal with that. My high school experience was so far removed from the average as to be frankly inapplicable to most. I was essentially in a single classroom that was qualified to give diplomas according to the government. We were all one or two cliques; there was none of the larger social environment that defined high school for most.

At this time, I should also note that Gateway was a school dedicated to autism and my autism was the far more central and in the limelight aspect of my life. In many ways, my autism pushed Marfan syndrome fully out of my mind. My life was defined by my neurological issues, not my heart or my back. At least, not until my senior year.

Something strange was going on in my senior year. Around that time, I was about 6'5". However, a few years before this, I was 6'6". I was shrinking. I ended up losing another inch before we got this straightened out. As a matter of fact, I was physically straightened.

This may all sound quite shocking, but we knew about this for a while before we had to deal with this. No surprise surgeries this time; something like that would not occur for about a decade. This process of shrinking happened over the course of my seventeenth and eighteenth years, finally climaxing when I was nineteen. We were forewarned and prepared. I did not have any fantasies about wishing this away or ignoring it. It was coming.

What we were preparing for was the severe scoliosis I developed in my late teens. Scoliosis is when the spine starts to collapse into itself and curve, usually taking an "S" or "C" shape. My spine was practically doing a "U" shape, taking a U-turn if you will. I said as much to my orthopedist when I saw my x-rays while this was happening. I told my doctor it looked like my spine was making a U-turn. That was why I was shrinking; my back was literally starting to collapse into itself. If something were not done to correct this, my spine and other organs would be subject to major injury, in the latter case because my spine would begin to pinch into my organs. Scoliosis only affects about 3% of the population last I checked, and mostly affects folks with conditions that cause people to grow tall faster than most. This is something people with Marfan need to keep an eye out for. The bottom line: this condition that was now upon me was a result of my Marfan syndrome.

Shortly after my nineteenth birthday, not long after Christmas (my birthday is in January), which was my marker for remembering all of this, we flew off once more to Baltimore. I remember when this happened quite clearly, because that Christmas, I got my first smart phone. Ironic that around the time my world changed so dramatically, so did the rest of the actual world. The Information Age was about to take steroids, and one of the single most dramatic decadal changes in culture was about to occur right alongside such a monumental change within my own life.

I remember that we pushed the surgery off just a tad as to allow me to enjoy both Christmas and my birthday; I believe Johns Hopkins wished to perform the surgery in either December or November of the year before. Obama had not been sworn in yet; I was recovering in Baltimore from the second most invasive surgery in my life, and at the time, the single most invasive surgery in my life, when he put his hand upon those bibles. What a thing to remember!

Once in Baltimore, much of it was second verse, same as the first. We checked into a hotel in the harbor area, The Four Seasons, the same one we had been going to every year when I flew in for my annual checkup. We would just enjoy ourselves for a few days before the time came, seeing movies and going to several fine seafood places. Then the day finally arrived. We got into a cab, my parents and I, and arrived at Johns Hopkins Hospital. We were then directed to where we would need to go to prep for anesthesia. There was no bizarre evil room this time, looking like something out of Robocop; it seems they had learned their lesson by this point and redecorated it!

I also received no potion this time, so no funny stories around that. I was far too old for that at this point. They simply prepped me with an IV, pumped me with saline a few times to test it (always a freaky feeling), and carted me off to the OR when it was time. While this was only my second surgery, this would become an unfortunately common routine over the next decade.

Then, the surgery happened. They made an incision from the base of my neck down to my waist while following my spinal column. Once this was accomplished, they straightened out my spine and kept it all in place with a Harrington Rod, a stainless-steel ratcheting rod used to correct spinal curvature invented by one Paul Harrington (thus the name) in 1959.

I was 6'4" when I went into the operating room. I came out of the OR 6'10".

Apparently, not only had my scoliosis caused me to shrink, but it had also stagnated my growth. Not that anyone had noticed at the time, with how fast I grew. It just ended up that I was growing even faster than we believed, but the curvature of my spine hid it. That little illusion was blown away when I grew six inches within the course of six or so hours, however long the surgery lasted.

Remember how I said this was only the second most invasive surgery in my life? Well, considering they full on manipulated and augmented my spinal column with surgical grafts, that should say a lot about what was to come. I should also note that it came with the longest recovery time. In most regards at least. While it took me a year to fully recover from this surgery, I was not actually hospitalized for all that long. Relatively speaking at least; certainly, three weeks is long by most standards, but I had my spine straightened out.

After I was checked out of the hospital, I was shipped back to the hotel, a portent of things to come. They put me into a van while in a wheelchair. A very padded, very comfy wheelchair, and I was on oxycontin. I hate to imagine how things would have been if not for the painkillers. This was indeed one of the single most painful moments in my life. At that point in my recovery, being in any position besides completely flat on my back was excruciating agony, pills and pillows be damned.

I remember trying to sit up in the hotel restaurant to have breakfast. We were trying to increase my endurance and I was hungry. I had to abort halfway through due to feeling like one of those poor souls who were tortured in the Tower of London during the height of its operation. There goes my creative mind again, but this time, a bit on the morbid side.

It was not all bad, as it allowed me to justify eating easy to eat, tasty finger foods like bacon and chicken tenders. I had bacon and toast meals regularly while we still were at the hotel. Considering what I had just gone through, it was a miracle that

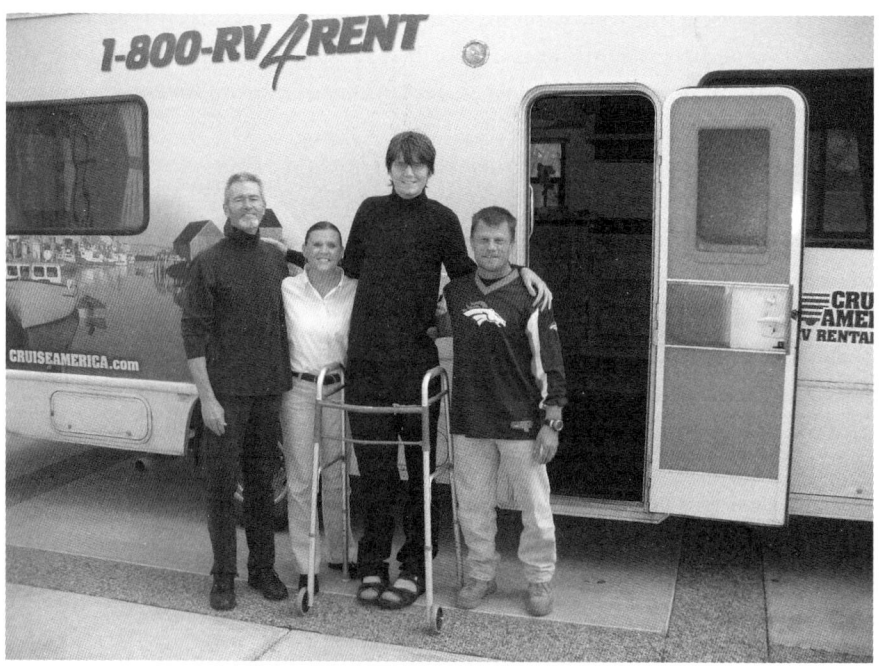

After 3 months in Johns Hopkins and a hotel room, I and my support crew successfully arrive home in Arizona from Baltimore after driving an RV for 4 days and through 13 states. My spinal surgery and 28-inch metal rod implants to correct scoliosis added five inches to my height but made flying impossible.

my digestive tract was completely unaffected so I could eat anything (even if most things, due to requiring me to sit up, were somewhat difficult to enjoy through the pain) and it really was a convenient food considering my condition. My parents did not get in the way of whatever I felt I wanted to eat because of everything I had been through. The hotel makes masterful bacon, by the way. Same with the toast. Tenders were merely acceptable.

John, my martial arts teacher and therapist, was not in the mood to just let my health slide like that. John had flown over to help with my recovery. For free in fact. My parents paid for his flight and his room, but he refused payment for his services here. He was doing this as my friend. At this point he was one of my best friends. He admits he came to see me as a surrogate little brother. He went about putting me through my paces, trying to get my endurance back to somewhat acceptable levels. Get me used to standing and walking and sitting again. Hopefully, trying to get me to the point where a five-hour plane ride would be tolerable and not horrific agony. Honestly, if we tried to leave when we first checked out of the hospital, I dare say the airline would have kicked us out before we even took off. There is no worse publicity for your services than someone screaming like they were in hell sitting in First Class and proceeding to do that for five hours. John did his best.

He was somewhat successful. I was able to tolerate sitting through a full meal. I also think I know what heaven feels like and it feels like the sheer relief I felt when I could finally lie down in my hotel bed. I was able to walk a fair distance with the help of my walker and stand up for a fair length of time. Standing and walking were easier for me than sitting was, probably because I got to keep my back straight. Still, while standing did not cause me nearly as much pain as sitting, it was physically exhausting, so I certainly was incapable of doing so indefinitely. Still, for all the progress John had made with me, the simple fact of the matter was that there was no way I could possibly tolerate a five-hour flight. My parents had no idea how we were going to get home, perhaps even thinking we would have to stay in Baltimore until I got well enough. That notion was quickly dismissed, as we had no idea how long it would take for me to tolerate such a trip (though based on what I know now, it would have taken a year). My parents were considering an expensive series of train trips when my Dad came upon a novel idea.

We would rent an RV with a sufficiently large bed, and then road trip from Baltimore all the way back to Paradise Valley, Arizona. All while I get to lie down through the whole thing. This was the option we ultimately settled upon. It was certainly quite the experience. I believe the trip took about 4 days, a little short of a week, with John and Dad (with Mom occasionally pitching in) trading off driving duties in shifts. I did not exactly get the opportunity to appreciate America as one should on these trips, what with being confined to bed and not really having a good view of the windows.

That does not mean I was completely denied the entire quintessential American road tripping experiences. Quite a few gas stations, McDonald's, and roadside diners were raided for food, and so I got to enjoy it all. I do believe we stopped at a tourist trap to take pictures. I cannot remember what giant T-Rex or giant rubber-band ball we stopped at, but I do have the group picture we took. Mom, Dad, and John were posing for the picture, with the now gargantuan Christopher smiling and struggling not to tip over. I felt like a dead redwood tree while clutching desperately at my walker. My smile was genuine though. What a sight we must have been.

John pulled a bit of a prank here. See, he has something of a reputation for being an absent-minded professor type. Thus, he played at having misplaced the RV key for just long enough for Dad to start to panic before pulling out the key. I remember clear as day what Dad said then, a strained smile upon his face. "John, you ass!"

Eventually we arrived back home in Arizona. I have no idea how we got the RV back to the rental agency; I think someone came and picked it up for us. Poor guy having to take that thing cross country for us.

It would take me a year to recover to something like full health, and about three years until I could say I regained everything lost that could be regained. I ended up getting back into school frankly a lot sooner than I think I should have. This was due to a combination of my own stubborn desire to graduate before twenty, and external pressures I cannot go into. It is not my place.

When I say go back to school, I do not mean physically. That would not happen until the second half of the semester. I would spend the first half of the school year working from home. Luckily, most of the curriculum was brought to me by my teacher, Patty Tusay, and we worked digitally as well. Honestly, I probably should have done the entire semester, but let us just say there were several stubborn people involved, including myself. So, I ended up back in the classrooms, such as they were, at Gateway Academy. To be honest, I was concerned how my peers would see me, but I should not have been afraid. They were all so caring. In fact, Julie commented, "When Chris had his surgery, I was hoping that it would help him, which it seemed it did. I kept thinking it must have been so hard now to be even taller and so limited." My friend Robert also said something similar; "Mostly glad to have my friend back, but also felt pity because the activities we easily could do together were not so easy anymore."

I was just recovered enough to tolerate sitting up for a full class period, but only just barely, and only if I could take frequent breaks to lie down. Thank God the chairs were comfy and allowed me to lean back so far as to practically render me flat on my back. I thank every God that has ever been dreamed of and those that had not for the abundance of beanbags throughout the building. Who knew that weird autistic thing that I never really bought into would end up helping me so greatly during my Marfan syndrome time of need?

Sadly, the limitations of Marfan syndrome finally caught up with me and could no longer just be ignored. I no longer could bend my back enough to touch my feet. I had to contort and do weird things to get dressed. For the longest time I wore nothing but sandals due to how easily I could slip them on without socks. I needed so much help, for things that were once second nature. However, some of these limitations hit an area I loved the most.

I could not fully devote myself to a sport I was passionate for due to my heart. A sport I could have excelled at, perhaps have even been world champion like my mentor, John. Instead, my passions cooled, and my advancement to Black Belt slowed to a crawl. I was now limited.

I could not deny it this time.

CHAPTER FIVE:
TRANSITIONS

There he was, the gentle giraffe, he who grazed upon the trees as easily as the gazelle grazed upon the plains. He was out-massed only by the venerable elephant, and yet he is still taller! The sheer force of his kicks makes even the mighty lions of the savannah think twice about approaching, but most importantly, there he stood, tall and proud! There was something wrong with this picture, because this giraffe was no longer standing, and would not for a good long while.

In fact, this giraffe was stuck flat on his back. God, imagine if we were not speaking of a metaphorical giraffe here, but rather the genuine article? The image is both very funny and very sad.

When I was flat on my back, I was still in high school. I had to ask for everything, and I was being watched very carefully. I was somewhat recovered, but still needed to take frequent walks and ask to go to the restroom to look for a flat surface or bench to lay upon to assuage the aches in my back. In contrast, in the first few years of college there were freedoms I was not accustomed to, and I became drunk with this newfound freedom. I made a lot of mistakes, but I think it was because I was so controlled in high school, I just needed to cut loose. However, by the time I was close to a full recovery, I was well established in the world of college. I still made mistakes, sometimes even epic ones, but no longer from inexperience or due to being overwhelmed by newfound freedom. I just had a terrible time with transitions.

I remember I gave the impression that I dove straight into homeschooling straight out of the RV. However, it was not that long after arriving home (I was obviously still living with my parents at the time) that schooling began. I am uncertain as to the exact amount of time I had to myself before I got back into the thick of things, but I do know it was at least a few weeks of no stress. I do call no school no stress.

I remember being absolutely glued to my television, something that had not been the case for a long time. My usual hobbies, the Internet and video gaming, required me to either lean forwards or sit up. At least they did in my case because I was so nearsighted.

I should clarify that when I say I was glued to my television, I meant my parents' television. My parents were set on spoiling me to make up for all the pain I was going through, so I spent much of my time lying upon my parents' far comfier bed. Besides which, my personal television was not actually for watching television, but purely for DVDs and gaming. No cable, no channels—merely a display screen.

I was not completely divorced from the Internet, as I had received my first smart phone (an iPhone 3G, the original model) the previous Christmas. I was incredibly grateful for this, as it saved me from soul crushing boredom while in Baltimore. However, I was still not used to the thing, so when I had other options, I tended to take them. Trying to view the World Wide Web through that tiny screen was not exactly the most comfortable thing but I made do.

I got very acquainted with the Cartoon Network during my time stuck at home, both during the time I was just convalescing and when I was being homeschooled. I admit that I started enjoying shows that, when I look back on them, were not all that good. When whatever on Cartoon Network was intolerable even with me at the time having a heightened tolerance for bad shows, I would start watching Animal Planet or the Discovery Channel. But really, I was just bored and lacking energy. I was unable to really sit up for any length of time. I made do with the choices I had. I guess you can call it making deals with myself. In many ways, this formed habits that frustrate me even to this day.

I was stuck flat on my back, that's for sure, and moving from one place to another was an exhausting (though much less so by that point) exercise of using my walker to get to one place or the other. I was also just constantly exhausted, so even when I found something active and fun I could do on my back, like handheld game consoles, such as the Nintendo DS and the PlayStation Portable/PSP or the nascent mobile gaming market popping up on smart phones, I often felt so low energy that I decided to pursue more passive forms of entertainment like television, reading, and Internet browsing.

I guess a parent might be thinking that reading more is not exactly a bad thing. First, please remember why your child is currently reading instead of playing video games. Yes, reading more may still be something seen as a silver lining, but I gained a habit of engaging in passive pursuits in general at the expense of active ones. Obviously, gaming is not the only active thing you can do, but this applies equally to other active pursuits like art or writing. For me, this led to the incredibly frustrating fact that, even though I have been studying literature and the art of writing for a decade, I only started actively writing in the last four or so years. I also believe that is the main reason (on top of the already mentioned frustration over not being able to compete in sparring tournaments) why my advancement in Tae Kwon Do slowed so drastically. The frustration of my situation led to bad habits that really slowed down my progress in the things I loved to do. I still trained during my scheduled training hours, once I was recovered enough for such things of course, and I put in 110% during those times, but I no longer practiced much outside of these scheduled hours like I used to.

However, right now, I want to talk about what my life was like when it was pretty much a blur of cartoons, animal/science shows, eating, physical therapy, and showers. Funny thing here is that showers, while I couldn't exactly luxuriate for hours on end in there, were one of the few sitting (as we obviously used a shower chair during this time; too risky otherwise) activities I could actually enjoy long term. My back still hurt, but the hot water soothed away the pain, at least to a point. Hot showers always felt extra amazing when I was recovering from a surgery. Baths pretty much stopped being a thing altogether from this point forward because I was now nigh seven feet in length and was unable to bend my back much at all. I literally could not and still cannot fit into normal sized bathtubs. At least if I wanted to clean anything above the waist. I need a Jacuzzi sized tub to take a bath and, frankly, showers are just easier. These are the things people with Marfan, like me, might have to deal with—the possibility of no baths. Does this seem trivial? Not if you like baths and want to be like others who are able to enjoy these things.

Eventually though, homeschooling would start. We were only going to do this for the first half of the semester. We really should have finished my last year this way. However, there were external pressures here, and I also stubbornly wanted to spend at least a part of my final year in high school on mandatory education with my school chums.

Luckily, the way Gateway Academy was structured, it made homeschooling easy. Most of our coursework was done via the Internet. We basically used a variety of programs designed for homeschooling already and combined that with a classroom setting and other projects and assignments. While I would miss out on any group projects, it was easy enough for the teachers and staff to fill in those credits with something equivalent, and beyond those few exceptions, they were able to give me whatever assignments that weren't in these programs over the phone or via e-mail.

My Gateway teachers were directly involved in this homeschooling. They would call me at mostly regularly scheduled times to communicate to me my course load for the day and get updates. Not all these times were convenient. I remember my English and Cultural Studies teacher, Patricia Tusay, coming to my house several times a week to help me finish the required literature courses so I could graduate. She was very thorough and friendly:

> Chris seemed happy to see me; I think boredom was starting to set in and being at home too much without his friends/peer contact was starting to be an issue. He was very bright and cheerful even with all he was going through. We settled into a routine and he did everything he needed to graduate which I feel was the greatest motivating factor to get back to school. (Patricia Tusay)

I did most of my work in bed via my laptop, but we made a point of at least doing the lecture bits sitting up and at the family desktop. Maybe this was ill advised, but we were trying to kill two birds with one stone here. That is, building up my endurance while also doing my schoolwork. It also helped prepare me for when I went back to school because there was no laptop and bed there. I was also allowed to rest whenever I needed to during these times. So much has become a blur with the timeline of events here, as they usually are for me.

Eventually the fated day arrived; I returned to school. I am sure my friends have plenty to say on that matter. Funny thing, though, is that I do not really remember it beyond "oh crud, this is going to be painful." This is because, ultimately, all the work had to be done sitting up and at a desktop.

I was always given the chair that was both the most stable and leaned back the most, and a healthy helping of pillows. Of course, with my nearsighted eyes, I still needed to get close enough to the screen to read anything. So, what often ended up happening is that I would be half lying off the table, or if no one was next to me, I would lie back in my chair and sit sideways and pulled physically as close to the desk as possible so that I was both leaning back and my face was close to the monitor. Then, when it came time to type, I would physically grab the keyboard and just type out whatever I needed to type while lying back, then lean forwards afterwards to see what needed fixing. I was quite creative. I am sure this annoyed some of the teachers and students at times.

Of course, even with all of that, I needed breaks to just be totally flat on my back and rest. I was given these breaks and I am so glad most autistic kids loved beanbags. I was never really one of them; mostly because my Marfan-syndrome-induced posture was not really accepting of sitting up in bean bags, but strangely this time, it worked. It meant easy access to places for me to just collapse and lie down. I was glad this too was just a part of transitioning to the next level when I would not have to do all these acrobatics to get through my day.

I technically only ended up graduating by the skin of my teeth. I say technically because I was an A and B student in almost all categories except one: Math. This would come to haunt me soon enough, but we will get to that. But graduate, I did! This was one of two graduations I felt were real; the other was my recent graduation from Arizona State University.

I intended to take a long break after this to just luxuriate in my adulthood. However, various factors were at work that caused me to start attending Scottsdale Community College in quick order. Strangely enough, I also intended to take a similar sabbatical after graduating from ASU. I wanted to spend 2020 chilling and traveling before I started cracking at my authorial career. The first bit was derailed quite quickly as I was contracted to write this book, which is far more fulfilling than my initial plans. The travel bit was also derailed for far less fortunate reasons, your basic pandemic which will most certainly be remembered as an historic event, one that pretty much shut down the planet. I again took this all in stride and went headlong into college, community college that is. I also wanted a different living situation while attending away from home.

At the very beginning, I stayed in a dorm specializing in special education, called Spectrum, with several of my high school classmates. I only stayed there for about two to three semesters before my parents and I decided that I should move back in with them for personal reasons. That lasted for about two years until I expressed interested in moving out. I was lucky to be funded for the most part, so all I needed was a roommate to split costs with, and I was able to maintain an apartment and then later a house while being a full-time student without a job. I am certain I would have lived with my parents a lot longer if not for this fact. As for the roommate issue, my mom had a dancing protégé who was seeking new employment outside of NYC, and thus mom essentially threw me at one of her dancers to keep tabs on me. That is how I met Liz Foldi. My roommate and I started with an apartment and moved to another apartment, before finally moving to the house we currently live in. This made going to college a lot easier, and funding was never an issue thanks to my family.

I spent my first four years at Scottsdale Community College. Eventually, I ended up pursuing my bachelor's degree for a whole decade due to all my past medical issues, but I was in a two-year program at SCC to get a head start in ASU when I transferred. Those previously mentioned medical issues/surgeries were things I could not avoid, but doubled the time needed to get an associate degree, this was all on me alone.

Remember how I said I barely scraped by in math? Well, that resulted in me having to take a lot of math classes. This was one of the reasons that I was there for four years. Scottsdale Community College is easily one of the biggest community colleges in the nation. When I say that, I am not talking the size of the student body (though that is quite large as well) or how successful it is. I mean literal size. It is pretty much a small town. It even has a central park. I guess it was about three miles from one end to the other, and do not ask me for square miles. This was going to be something of an issue, but not as much as you are likely thinking it is. After all, as I said prior, I was actually pretty good at walking.

In fact, I did a lot of walking in the first few years after my back surgery. As I have noted, I have a lot of nervous energy, and I should clarify that, when I say nervous energy, I do not mean I'm always nervous about something so much as I am restless when thinking or emotional. I tend to pace a lot when I am thinking over things. Some attribute this to autism and others to ADD/ADHD. Whichever it was, I had it. As previously stated during my recovery, standing up brought a lot less pain than sitting down, and this held true even a few years after the surgery. If you combine this with the nervous energy, I often found myself taking short walks after the pain of sitting down got a bit too much. I should note that when I say pain, I do not mean the hellish agony I felt immediately after the surgery nor even the "mere" pain from my final year as a high school student. It was a progressive backache that was quite tolerable if I must tolerate it, even though I'd just rather not. I had to take care of alleviating these issues.

The best part about college was that one does not need to ask permission to do this. For some students this could risk them losing attendance credits, and I will not pretend that this never was a risk for me. I reduced the amount of "bathroom breaks" I took by quite a bit after being told that misusing my medical condition to essentially skip class while technically not playing hooky could hurt my grades. After failing a course that I really should not have failed due to attendance (or more accurately the lack thereof), I took this to heart. I still took a lot of breaks, but now, they were actually breaks and not me arriving to class to sign in and then going to the "restroom" for half the class. I had a friend describe this as upgrading from felon to hooligan. I did acquire a bit of an attitude at SCC regarding my class attendance. My attitude led me to doing something quite monumentally stupid.

I am sure that I was not the only one with this issue when making the initial transition from mandatory K-12 education to college. I probably had it a bit worse because the student body at Gateway was so very small that teachers could afford to micromanage us to an even greater degree than is typical of a regular public high school. Regardless, all high school students must deal with a lot more structure and administrative interference than they ever do in college.

The sudden freedom was, frankly, a shock. I could skip a class without getting sent to the principal's office. Perhaps this is too generous as it implies that I even could skip class if I were willing to deal with the consequences. In high school, my movements were way too tightly controlled for that ever to be the case; I was driven to school and back, and my teachers shuttled me from class to class. The closest I could ever get to playing hooky during high school was surfing message boards and the Internet in general when I was supposed to be working on school assignments, but I was still in class. As for just going to the bathroom, you still needed to raise your hand and ask for permission.

Therefore, suddenly having the freedom to just not attend and leave the classroom whenever I pleased, unless it was pointed out I was being disruptive, was intoxicating during my first year. This led to me starting to form some bad habits in my first semester, but a combination of factors stopped me from going all out and self-sabotaging until the second semester.

First, pretty much all the classes I selected were things I had great interest in, like ancient mythology and writing, and I went to class because I wanted to. I found them entertaining and for the classes where this did not apply, my old high school instincts kept me from going all out with my newfound freedom. There was a voice in the back of my mind telling me to be cautious in case they decided to pull the rug out from under me and reveal that it was high school all over again and I just fell for their trap.

Yet, I still indulged in this new freedom to a point and got nothing but As and Bs once the semester was through. The fact that I got these after spending several days on campus just playing video games and eating and not attending any classes combined with what looked like loitering on campus was a bit crazy. However, it did empower me to fall on my face as I, in retrospect, began preparations to make an absolute ass of myself the following semester.

One of the classes I took was a computer science class. Oddly enough, I was better with computers back then than I am nowadays. Back then, I had some aspirations of being a programmer. I always intended to write creatively, do not mistake me, but back then I mostly wanted to do it via interactive stories, visual novels, and story heavy video games. I studied computers in pursuit of this goal. Ultimately, I figured out that I had no head for numbers, even if I had a pretty good head for theory, so I ultimately let it drop. Do you want me to be honest? The result of all this was that I aced the final exam for computer science and still managed to fail the class because I skipped out on a quarter of my classes and only did half the homework. Interesting fact I learned at SCC was that missing homework does not automatically get you the teacher's ire; this was also a hell of a change for me. It was not a positive experience, but a rude awakening to say the least.

While a lot of this was due to my immaturity and personal failings at the time (not shifting the blame), I can't help but think that my then current medical woes did not play at least some small part in my lackadaisical attitude towards school. I did talk at length about the pain I was going through and my lack of energy. Well, this also translated into generally decreased motivation to do much of anything beyond lie down and surf the web and play video games. More the former than the latter to my ongoing frustration. Those bad habits were coming back to bite me. Again, not looking to shift the blame, but classes were physically exhausting and, at times, flat out painful. Eventually, I learned that I could nap in the shade of the trees in the central park area or read a book while lying down upon a couch in the lounge instead of going to class without immediately getting into trouble.

OK, so I had a lot of temptation is what I am trying to say. None of that excuses skipping so many classes and homework assignments that even getting a 100 on my final exam still could not save me from a failing grade. But it does tie into my physical challenges. Eventually, I got to the point where I had recovered from my back operation as much as physically possible without replacing my spine with something from the TV show, *Six Million Dollar Man*. I had a lot more transitions and schooling ahead of me.

CHAPTER SIX:
IS THIS MY LIFE?

Skipping classes and homework assignments and failing a class was the culmination of all my horrible academic habits. This was because I got drunk upon my newfound freedom. And yet, every other class I had during that first year, other than the one I failed, I received nothing but As and Bs.

Now, much of that was because I was exclusively taking classes that I was interested in at the exclusion of any of those boring prerequisites. Computer science (that is, the class that I failed) was a class I thought would qualify as one of those fun courses when I selected it. As I said, I had some illusions about becoming a programmer on top of being a writer back then. I wanted to focus on my storytelling talents mostly within the medium of video games. I still do wish to write for some games, but it is no longer my primary focus. I really do not have the head for programming based on my limited math skills. I learned that if I was not interested in it (or lacked the skills for it, but that applies to everyone), the greater the chance I failed it. Therefore, it was my fun courses which allowed all those As and Bs during my first year of truancy and delinquency. But it certainly was not the only or even primary reason I got these good grades.

The unsung heroes, or as some less charitable souls may call enablers in this circumstance, in all of this is the DRS of SCC (Disability Resource Services office of Scottsdale Community College). Their job is what it says upon the tin; they manage accommodations for those with various disabilities. While they try to individualize these accommodations to each unique case, we got a large selection of standardized accommodations. Not that we usually needed much beyond this standard set: they were quite robust. Everything from extended test time to paperwork authorizing students to bring in specialized medical equipment. They were prepared for almost any circumstance and could easily adapt in times when needed. They were also exceedingly easy to utilize. Just go in, present truth/documentation of your disability, explain what you need, sign a bit of paperwork, and they will file folders for all the relevant teachers and accommodations and off you go! I won't dwell upon this here, as this is more relevant to the parts of the book covering my time at Arizona State University, but the service at SCC was so much better than their equivalents at ASU for this reason alone. ASU required all of it be done digitally, and their website was a finicky mistress.

The reason I said that some may call them my enablers in that first year, is that I went whole hog on accommodations that first year. After all, I had just recovered from the second most invasive surgery in my life, so why wouldn't I? Much of this resulted in what I believe to be too much leeway from teachers. However, some of those file folders had accommodations that explicitly said that I may need to leave class for periods at a time due to pain, so please accommodate.

After that first year (and a bit into the second), I only dealt with three accommodations. One was for notetaking. One student in whatever class I was in, and had those accommodations for, would be paid around $40 a class once for a semester and they would give me copies of their notes. They were supposed to do this by taking notes on specially designed copy paper provided by DRS. Not all did this. Usually, they would e-mail me photos of their notes or photocopy their notes. The other accommodations that I regularly employed were for test taking. These translated into extended testing time and providing a scribe to make up for my slow writing speed. You might notice something of a pattern with these. They seem to be accommodations for my autism and ADD, and not my Marfan syndrome. That is because, once more, this next chunk of my life was defined more by my various neurological issues than the bevy of physiological issues that stem from my Marfan syndrome. At least, once I had finished my recovery from my spinal surgery, I still took frequent walks to help deal with back pain, just not to an excessive degree. This was important as the teachers did not question me and just assumed I had a weak bladder (what helps is that I do, in fact, have one). That was about it at this point as far as accommodations from the staff were concerned. The rest of my Marfan-related needs, like securing comfy seats at the café and making sure I had enough leg room during classes, were something I took care of on my own.

I remember Patricia Tusay (Patty), my tutor and academic advisor, would often push me to grab more accommodations than I already had. "Grab every advantage you are entitled to Chris, even if you don't need them at that moment," she would say. "No such thing as an unfair advantage if you have a disability." This is not exploiting the system, and it extended to accommodations for my physical ailments as well. I remember one time both Patty and DRS pushed for me to get this customizable desk thing so I would not have to crane my neck as much as I do, but lugging that thing around just seemed like more trouble than it was worth. Not every accommodation worked out.

I would try out a number of these suggestions from Patty and DRS, of course, but inevitably I would return to the usual core notetaker plus test accommodations. At the end of the day, it's infinitely easier to go to the teacher and give them the paperwork needed for the test accommodations and get a notetaker than to ask them to set up my own personal tech support team and other overcomplicated ideas and equipment.

The overall point of all this is to say, for the next few years, my Marfan syndrome took a backseat to my neurological issues, but not because they were easy to ignore like before. The back pain never quite went away, and I was forever incapable of fully bending my back.

I could not ignore it, but for the time being everything that could be done had been done.

All that was left was to adapt and to endure. I was good at that. Almost too good at that.

I learned to get into cars without arousing too much attention, and how to close the car door with my foot. I also learned how to look a bit smug while doing it, so that people would assume that I do it for style points and not because I needed to do this. I would rather folks think I was some Han Solo like lovable jerk, and not an object of pity. There were a few adjustments to be made along the way.

Socks also went out for the next five or so years, as I could not put them on without help. Thus, they only came out when I needed to wear fancy shoes for fancy events. Sandals and slip-on shoes were the order of the day, and that is only when I needed to leave the house. Indoors (or even in my own backyard), my feet were bare as the day I was born. However, they would not stay as smooth as the day I was born, and this would cause me no end of problems years later.

Perhaps the adaptation that frustrated me the most was the fact that if I was not doing anything important, my immediate instinct was to find a couch or bed and lie down. I am pretty sure I have been flat on my back for more than 50% of my life at this point. What makes this so darn frustrating is that activities like writing and video games are suddenly things I needed to hype myself up for! Gaming used to be my default state, not something special, but once sitting up became a light workout, there was hesitation. But these were things I did for myself, not things others did for me. I mean, obviously those in the know did what they could, like help putting on my socks and helping me get out of cars. But my physiological issues, even if they no longer could be just ignored, were once again not at the forefront of my mind. This was something to endure until the next batch of surgeries a few years later.

My circle of friends and my living situation drastically changed during this period, and you will need to know who Liz is and when I moved into my own place. For this, I want to return to my first year in college. I spent about a year at Spectrum. It was actually run by the administration of Gateway Academy, and I stayed there with several of my old high school classmates. The sales pitch for the place was support staff for our various conditions, as well as counseling and therapy while attending some type of post-secondary education program.

For that first year, things were rather good. It was when the staff was rotated out the next year, problems started. I do not wish to resurrect old, personal dramas, so let us just say the new staff was less than capable, and I was pulled out by my parents. For the next year I lived with my parents. Things were pretty much as they were when I was a teenager growing up with them. My dad woke me up at 10 AM at the latest regardless of what was happening that day. School day, or a completely free day, dad was consistent. Small breakfast and lunch because I never had an appetite at those times due to my ADHD meds, and big dinners because suddenly I was STARVING now that the pills had worn off. My parents would drive me to school and back. It was no different from how things were when I was going to high school, only with a slightly different schedule and school, and frankly I wanted out of that. College was supposed to be different. I wondered how my parents felt about my being at home at this age, so I asked my dad:

> Speaking of Spectrum, in that time you, you know, you grew up a lot. You know, the normal growing up process. I found you were definitely more mature, and I think the fact that you were suddenly for the first time in your life really living outside of our, then your, home... look, any time but I think people do that, it forces you to expand your horizons, think about things differently, suddenly you're having to deal with well, that would cause anyone to grow up! But you know I think you just living on your own and not with us forced you to think about things differently. It becomes very comfortable when you're living with your parents all the time, and when you're sort of outside your comfort zone in your life, I do think it makes you expand your horizons just a little bit. (At Spectrum) you had to deal with new people, day in and day out, and that expands your vocabulary as you hear the new words they are using! You became a little more self-sufficient. With me and mom you just expect us to do everything, because we are so used to doing everything for you, and I am assuming you knew that. When you are suddenly in an environment where they were expecting you to do a lot more for yourself. I believe they had you making your bed or whatever. When you came back you were just, you're more mature you were a little

more self-sufficient and you use new words new thoughts from dealing with all these new people in your life it expanded your horizons quite a bit. I was sad to see you go because I love having you at home. I have a feeling that's kind of normal for any parent, you know. You hate to see your kids go, to see them grow up and no longer be a kid. Yet at the same time that's exactly what you want them to do; to go out and fly on their own, if I can use a bird analogy for a second, to see YOU flying out on your own. But I was sad to see you go, but I also had a feeling that you were very prepared to do that. I was really concerned of course, as you have a lot of medical issues and I was worried about things like are you going to take your pills every day because I was always there every day to make sure that happens. So, I was concerned about that, but I also thought you were prepared to do that on your own, and I also knew you were going to be with Lizzy right? So, there was someone who could keep an eye on you. Even if it was not me or your mom. (Peter Talbert)

Peter continued to talk about how I was as an adult tenant in the household:

As you know, when before you went to Spectrum, I felt you often liked to argue, you were like a lawyer, and I would often find that you will take positions I wasn't really sure you believed in, but it was almost like you just want to argue. Whereas, when you came back as an adult, you still had positions, but they are much more thought out, thoughtful, and more... more in line with what you really believe as opposed to just wanting to be the devil's advocate. (Peter Talbert)

I petitioned for an apartment of my own to live in, primarily to my mom. She likes to spoil me, but she was scared out of her mind with just throwing me out there on my own. Thankfully, a friend of hers, a former dancer (now massage therapist) by the name of Liz Foldi, was looking to move out of New York to one of the resort states. Looking after me a bit was good work for her skillset now that she was no longer dancing. In short, mom threw me at one of her dancers to take care of me.

In many ways, this is an incredibly unfair assessment of the situation, especially given what I now know of Liz Foldi and how our relationship progressed. Liz did not uproot her whole life and move to another state because Ann Reinking decreed it. She was going to move regardless, and Arizona was one of many of her options, and mom simply took the opportunity and narrowed it down for her former protégé. It certainly does not apply to my second roommate, Barbara Sause, who might be able to make her equines dance, but was never one of mom's dancers.

Yet the simple fact remains; I doubt mom would have helped finance me moving out if not for Liz being there. At first, it really did feel like I was still living with my parents, just with a middle-aged woman. Especially considering for the first few years in my new apartment, like clockwork, I went back to my parents' place for every weekend and holiday.

It was in a nice little gated condominium complex called Aderra. Two bedrooms, two bathrooms, a large combination living room and kitchen area, it was definitely a nice place.

I did mention this technically being my second place as well. Well, let us just say that we did not fully read the fine text when we leased the place. We had assumed that it was the next best thing to outright buying the place. We did not have to pay rent, we got a discount, and the place simply reverted to them if we moved out so we would not need to deal with selling the place. Of course, that also meant we could not sell the place either, because it was not entirely ours, but things were already a bit too good to be true and it did remove a bit of hassle. We also thought we could not just be evicted. Apparently, that only applied to other leasers and those seeking to rent. But what if someone decided to buy the place outright?

Well, as you can probably guess by now, that is exactly what happened. It was quite the rude awakening. We moved elsewhere in the same complex, but this time we outright bought the place so that there could be no repeat of this debacle. It was identical to the first place, enough so that my memories have absolutely no way of distinguishing the time I was in the first place and the second place. As you recall, I have problems with sequential anything and details of events in order, so this is consistent. Therefore, I will be treating them as functionally the same location. I will say the second place had the superior view; we could only see the rest of the complex from the balcony of our first apartment, whereas we got an excellent view of the attached golf course and park area from the (structurally identical) balcony of the second.

One of the best things about this Aderra complex location is that the neighborhood had everything needed within walking distance. For one, it encouraged me to work out on my own as I walked to several locations, and two, it allowed me a far greater feeling of independence in a time where that feeling was lacking. Subway, gas stations, McDonald's, Chipotle, IHOP, multiple video game stores, supermarkets, and restaurants of a dizzying variety were at my feet. The sky seemed to be the limit to a young man who was used to mom and dad and an army of nannies and caretakers taking me everywhere. Also, everything was at least a half-mile walk away, so it was good exercise.

Now that we have the new location situated within your collective minds, let us talk for a bit about the person I was sharing this new living space with…Liz Foldi. Obviously, this is not her biography, and frankly it is not my place to divulge all that I know, but I will tell you a little something about her.

Liz met mom when Liz was only twelve. She was a young dance student who caught my mom's eye, especially when they all got cast into various roles in the film *All That Jazz*. Mom was Liz's mentor, both in dance and elsewise during the production of that film. The mentor/protégé relationship continued long past the completion of that production. When Liz came of age, she would eventually follow mom onto Broadway.

Another important thing to remember about Foldi is that she is intensely religious, a Born-Again Christian. She was raised Catholic, but something personal happened, and she converted. Luckily, she is no zealot, so the most that this affected my life was that I was now surrounded in well-worn bibles and religious artifacts and artwork, along with the occasional theological discussion. However, my second roommate, Barbara, was a lot more intense when she came into my life. She, like Liz, was hardcore religious, but no real inconvenience for me. She is Liz's friend.

As for the reason Liz moved to our beautiful state of hundred-degree weather and open carry, she had another passion other than dance and Jesus. One that she devoted herself to full time once she retired from the dancing world, and that was massage therapy. Work in that field was starting to dry up in New York. She needed to move, and mom made the "where" in that question easy. Yet more importantly than even work, however, is the matter of her parents. They were both retired and living in South Carolina. They increasingly needed more and more assistance from their daughter, so moving from New York was an inevitability due to that alone. Moving to Arizona and then moving her parents here as well was the optimum solution for her, as there was more work for her here than in South Carolina. But if they did not want to move here, Liz would have moved to South Carolina instead and I would have been down a roomie. Thankfully, it seems her parents found that the desert agreed with them. The rest, as they say, is history. I had roommates!

Now, some of you may well be wondering what my social situation was like outside of my family, roommates, and academic/professional acquaintances. Robert, if you remember him from earlier, was still around. He was great fun to have around, and he seems to agree:

> My thoughts were simply clear, concise, and straightforward. Having fun with my friend in a new environment where we had more control over our lives. The transition from high school to college was fresh early on with many mistakes. But I felt that those minor mistakes we fussed over were done on our own volition to really support ourselves mentally on where we wanted to go in life and what would be working best. You, yourself were no different from many others at SCC, as well as I. A milestone for us all with wildly different paths, and your path was

much more focused than others if I had to pinpoint something different about it all. (Robert)

For the first year, however, it really was just Robert and Eric (another fellow schoolmate from Gateway), and maybe one weird kid in the cafeteria that occasionally hit me up to discuss video games. Usually about the *Kingdom Hearts* series. Funny that I could remember our conversations, but not his name. That extends to my time in Spectrum. Yes, I was living with others 24/7 but really, I did not like anybody there, and that is all I will say on this matter.

That changed sometime in the second year. Somebody started hooking up video game consoles in the lounge area. This would result in spontaneous *Smash Bros* tournaments, and then this resulted in the same group of people gathering in the same location again and again. That included Robert. Eventually, we started to get in trouble for these gatherings. They said we were monopolizing the area. Did we back down? No.

Someone had the brilliant idea to legitimize our monopolizing the area. Thus, the Electronics and Games Club was formed, and we would designate the lounge area as our club meeting place. This group of fellow gaming nerds became my main source of a social life throughout my tenure at SCC, until its rather dramatic disbandment in the last year of my time there. But such stories will have to wait for just a little bit. However, when talking to Robert on the subject of this book in general, and this group in particular, he warned me against going further on this subject, "No. I am sorry, but I will have to refuse answering this one, as well as strongly recommend as your friend to not include that particular aspect of your higher education. I personally feel it has absolutely zero relevancy to your condition. Sorry."

It is funny really, how the mind can cause you to forget the unpleasant aspects of reality, of your past, and simply focus upon the pleasant. The more Robert and I spoke on the matter, the more I realized that he was probably right. However, he is not writing this book now, is he? True, some things are best left untouched, especially if they are unrelated to the topic at hand. However, the point was that I had a social life, and an example of a coping mechanism in action so I will tell my story.

Now, many of the details escape me, particularly when it comes to names. Funny that, seeing as these people made up a good majority of my social life back then. It probably shows just how little of a real impression they made upon me as individuals. They sure left an impression upon me as a group, particularly in the matter of the disbandment of our club. We stuck together to nerd out and feel like we belong, and not really to form long-term relationships. Fairweather friends of a sort.

I remember the official leader constantly trying to get us to be a proper club, but frankly the only reason he was our "leader" was because he was good at talking with the administration and the staff. He had no force of personality really, no presence or charisma, so beyond gathering where and when he said we should (and even then, mostly because that's what the administration told him we had to do), we did not really listen to him. I mean, when he set up *Smash Bros* tournaments, we were certainly game, but that is because that is something we just enjoyed doing anyways. He was very much the image of the beetle-like IT department drone, round without being noticeably obese, short but not too short, nerdy looking (glasses, messy hair, freckles, and acne) but generically so. Absolutely unremarkable looking in every way... which ironically was remarkable in its own right! If you have ever bought anything from a video game store, then you have probably seen a thousand of him already. The cherry on top of everything else is that he also demanded we pay him $20 up front for "gas" whenever any of us needed to carpool with him, though honestly, in hindsight, he was taking us for a ride and not just in his car. Just from this, you can see the cracks forming.

A few others I remember with some clarity is a wheelchair-bound fellow who I got into frequent debates about video games with. I remember asking if he wanted robot legs, and he asked me if I wanted to lose a foot off my legs in retaliation. I almost told him that yeah, losing a foot would make fitting into showers easier and would result in less lumps on my head, but I do not believe he would have appreciated that. There was a larger Asian fellow who was quite nice, and I believe still hangs out with Robert. The last one from that group who still does, after the implosion of said group. There was a tall and bulky glass of water who lived in a trailer in his parents' backyard (I knew this because he invited us all over for his birthday once) who was pretty much the poster child for "person who would and should be a student at Gateway Academy and/or The Child School/Legacy High School." The last person I remember with any clarity was a certain tomboy with an incredibly volatile temper and a chip on her shoulder the size of me, and she's going to end up being something of an important figure soon. One of her outbursts is what resulted in the forced disbandment of the club.

Our usual routine would be to just gather at the lounge area, hook up some consoles, and then just talk about whatever came to our minds. Often video games, sometimes whatever weird conflict or drama would pop up. Which, if you read over the descriptions of the average club member (kind of mentally out there), was often quite frequent and quite petty. A particularly awkward memory involved a feminist and trans member of our group in an argument, with the feminist telling the other they do not understand what being a girl was like, only for them to shout at the top of their lungs "I AM A GIRL!" All conversation in the club area immediately ceased, all games paused, and the awkwardness was absolute and so palpable that we could have spread it on toast. It was particularly awkward because the trans individual in question had barely begun transitioning and was still quite visibly (and most certainly audibly) male.

As stated before, while our intrepid leader tried constantly to engage in scheduled club activities, he was only ever even remotely successful when it came to game tournaments. We mostly just did whatever came to us. After all, this whole "club" only existed to legitimize, on paper, our monopoly over the lounge area during our club times. This would ultimately come back to bite us in the backsides... and cause our dissolution. Yet, that is a story that happens within my last years at SCC, and thus a story that must wait for just a little bit longer.

We are now moving onto my last years in SCC, what happened during that time, and my graduation from SCC and of ASU. Yet most importantly, we will talk about the absolute marathon of tests and surgeries that would define the next few years of my life.

CHAPTER SEVEN:
OPERATIONS DU JOUR

"How is my life progressing?" the giraffe asks of himself, staring into his reflection upon the watering hole, as his "friend" group merrily ignores his woes as they discussed all sorts of nonsense. Only Hyena really seemed to care, and he had his own problems. It is a question that I begin to ask myself more and more as we move into my second decade upon this earth. This is not an unusual question for a young man in college to ask himself. However, I differ in that it isn't the destination I am anxious about. Unlike pretty much every other college student asking themselves that question, I always knew where I wanted to end up, even if it has changed a tad. Yes, I had flights of fancy about growing up to be an astrophysicist or a quantum physicist, but in the end my heart always belonged to the written word. This may be a cliché, but for me, it is my truth.

What has made me ask these questions is what my journey has been so far. This is because my wheels just seem to be spinning in place on the road to this final goal. I admit, even though I knew intellectually I was in a better place than most, I sometimes envied those who were lost on that proverbial road. After all, being lost implies some manner of movement, even if in the wrong direction. I felt like I was just stuck in place.

"So where am I really headed?" I repeatedly asked myself this question. Now, there are many reasons for all this running in place, or perhaps more accurately, the sensation of running in place. After all, I did move forward, just at such a snail's pace that it often felt like I was wasting my time. Perhaps it was something else that kept me spinning that I tried to put out of my mind on top of others: Marfan.

Much of the fault for this lies squarely in factors beyond my control, some that I have already spoken about, and others that I will continue to discuss and explore.

There are indeed involuntary roadblocks. However, there are also roadblocks of my own foolish design.

My lack of energy resulting in a somewhat slothful attitude and a horrible procrastination habit has contributed to my being the hamster on the wheel in my life as well as my endless academic loop. It seems I was perpetually stalled in school and out of the work force but there was absolutely nothing but myself preventing me from engaging in personal writing projects to at the very least get myself out there at least on the Internet. Indeed, I made a few half-hearted attempts at starting such projects before my own ambitions intimidated me and I fell back on laziness. I am glad to say that nowadays, I at the very least have this aspect of my personality under some control. I have pushed the hamster off the wheel and on a treadmill. Yet, that is me blaming a vague attitude/behavioral problem. I also made one far more concrete mistake.

I first obtained an associate's degree from SCC (Scottsdale Community College) before getting my bachelor's degree. This was to make my academic journey easier. The SCC degree had a great deal of math credits needed to qualify. Correction, the degree only required one particular math course. However, that course had a slew of prerequisites that needed to be addressed in sequence. The smart thing to do here would have been to sprinkle these math courses into my schedule alongside other, more interesting courses, over my tenure at SCC. Sadly, I left them all to the end. I had already completed every course required for the associate's degree. Sadly, these math courses (three) needed to be done one after the other, and then I would have to finally do the required one. I created my own academic loop and kept spinning those wheels.

That translated into two years artificially added to my time at SCC, taking only one class per semester until I could finally take the math course I needed to graduate! It was quite embarrassing, realizing the pickle I had landed myself in. There I was, wanting to do anything other than math, but wound up doing nothing but math for too long. This was all my doing. That was not the case with the other stuff that held me back.

My medical issues and the surgeries I needed at the time also contributed to my being stuck in one place. Those afflicted with Marfan syndrome deal with malformations in their skeletal structure. Usually when one talks about the skeletal issues that come from Marfan syndrome, the spinal column is what comes up most often. After that, the hands and wrists often become a talking point, usually in the context of identifying if one potentially has the genetic condition as opposed to being a danger in and of itself. Also, those with Marfan syndrome tend to be flat footed as well. Of course, surgeries are needed to correct these issues and I was no exception.

Obviously, my spine was always a huge issue throughout my life, and of the skeletal issues one could have, issues with the spine have the most potential dangers.

After all, I had to get invasive reconstructive surgery to deal with my own spinal issues. Has my spine entirely left the picture even now, as will become quickly apparent? No. No it has not.

Marfan syndrome affects the whole skeleton to some degree. How this manifests and in what degree, varies for each Marfan patient. However, as aforementioned, my ankles and knees have always been an issue. In the case of the ankles, almost as big of an issue, at least in terms of how it affected my lifestyle, as my spine. It might not threaten my life the way the extreme curvature of my spine did, but it sure has a negative effect on how I live my life.

You see, my ankles, especially my right ankle, were a bit too large, and more importantly caused my foot to land at an unnatural angle. I was essentially walking on the sides of my feet to some degree or the other. As you can imagine, this resulted in a lot of issues, and a lot of pain, while walking. It should be noted that there really is a fair difference between how this manifested in both my ankles. In my left foot, this would result in my foot landing side first before ultimately flattening into a normal footfall. When it came to my right foot however, I did not just land side first, I stood on the side of my foot unless I consciously flattened my foot. Eventually, I could not even manage that. It was a progressive issue.

When it got too bad, that was the impetus for my parents to arrange for me to get a whole set of reconstructive surgeries, and not just for my right ankle. There were several things we needed to do eventually but weren't pressing that had to do with issues skeletal. Our doctors at Johns Hopkins recommended that seeing as we needed to go in for my ankle, we may as well get these other things done as well.

For one, the work done on my spine needed some minor readjustments: A proverbial tightening of the screws as it were. There was also my right kneecap, which had once gotten detached when I was much younger, which meant it had needed replacement for a while now. It just was not pressing. There was also to be a procedure on my hips and my shins as a necessary consequence of all the other surgeries, to ensure that my right leg was stable. This seems par for the course with Marfan especially with the common features we seem to share. According to my doctor, Paul Sponseller, "Typical features are tall stature, curved sternum, spinal curvature, long thin limbs, and flat feet. You are typical in most respects, but your feet are high-arched rather than flat." I was very happy that this was an experienced man for my surgery, "I have performed spinal fusion with rods, and foot reconstructions," he assured me. However, I was not happy with what was about to happen.

We flew into Baltimore once more, during the summer of 2010, for the surgery. I was actually quite surprised when my mother reminded me of the year of the procedure. I had thought it was later than that, and not a mere two years after my first spinal surgery. I swore I had a longer reprieve from constant surgeries than that.

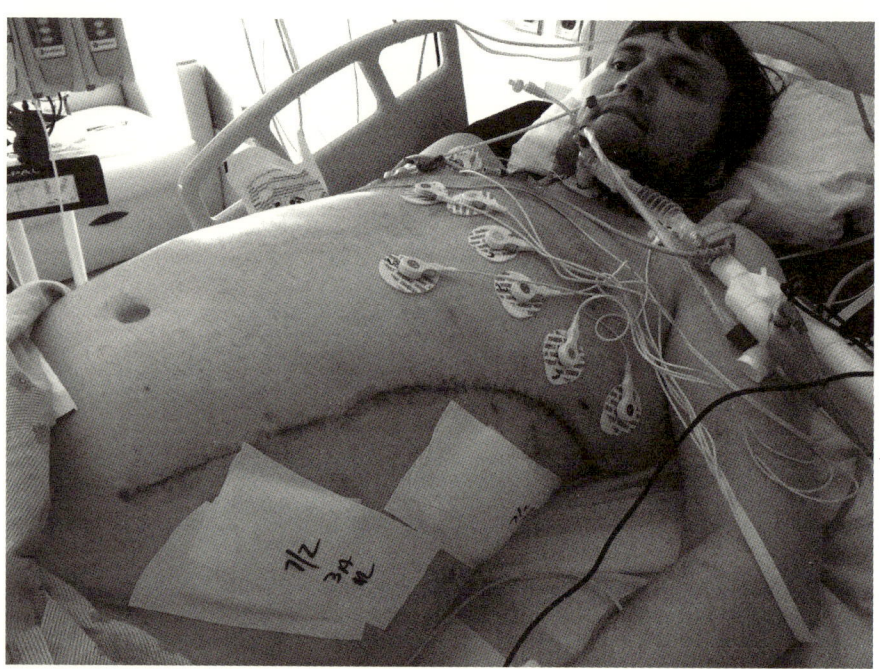

The second heart surgery which required an almost 4-foot incision from just below the nape of my neck around my side to just above my left groin. I like to tell people I survived a shark attack.

What I and my family did while in Baltimore waiting for the surgeries was the same as the time before that, or the time before that. Honestly, even most of my initial recovery was for the most part unmemorable. I was stuck in the hotel for a month, either stuck in bed or in a wheelchair. Which thankfully was not a literal torture implement this time around, despite the work done on the spine. Said work was very minor by comparison to what happened the last time I came to Baltimore for surgery, and so most of my irritation came from my right leg and my general immobility. Irritation was the right word for it, but we will get back to that in a second, as I do have one memorable story and a warning to give.

From my experience, do not check yourself/your loved one into a third-party recovery center, as they tend to be less skilled and less equipped. Try staying at the hospital till you/your loved one is okay enough to return home for the rest of the recovery. In my case, it was back to my hotel suite. It was the first time I was ever forced to deal with a bedpan, despite effectively only dealing with a broken leg. Apparently, everyone at this location (this place was recommended by my doctors) checked out at night and could not help me get to the restroom. I still do not understand why my doctors, usually very capable competent folks, would recommend to my parents that I should stay at this place for any number of days at all. Personally, I cannot help but feel as if they were using me as some sort of guinea pig for the viability of such locations. I hope the fact I got food poisoning at this location clued them in, because this course of action was never again suggested to us.

Yes, food poisoning. There was a cafeteria in this place that made really good sandwiches, but apparently their oversight was not the best. One sandwich my parents grabbed for me from the place had a rotten tomato in it. I was sick to my stomach nearly none stop for about two days. I did not need this on top of the pain I was having.

The pain I felt was never as bad as it was during my first spinal surgery, but due to just how much work was done during the surgery to my entire skeleton; my whole body felt a constant low level irritation; pins and needles and little aches all around. In a strange way, that made things worse than genuine pain, at least as far as my mood and temperament were concerned. I've been told before that I am the sort to become a stoic rock when tragedy strikes, yet whine like a babe when I spilled milk. It is like that here. Agony often prompts me to courageous stoicism. Mere irritation, on the other hand, prompts moodiness, surliness, and the abandonment of my good manners.

"Hold up," you say to the giraffe. "Irritation? Just irritation? They surgically implanted a small hardware store worth of metal into your legs and hips, on top of yet another spinal surgery! I can buy the first spinal surgery being worse, but that should be more than just irritation!"

The giraffe snorts in response. "Yes, I know I am very dismissive of what many would consider abject torment. Yet, I have had to deal with so much pain in my life that if I did not have such a skewed standard for pain, I am certain I would have gone insane by now. Now let's end this somewhat awkward use of the giraffe and get back to the story at hand."

That meant that I was less than pleasant company over the next two months. The first month was spent recovering and wheelchair bound in Baltimore, the second at my Aunt Jan and Uncle Dick's place in Washington State. The fact that my best friend Tommy joined me in Washington for the last week only slightly improved my mood.

I realize looking back that it is highly unlikely that what happened next was entirely the fault of my admittedly crap behavior and not just the straw that broke the camel's back on a mountain of stresses Mom was under since the surgery. Nevertheless, while I am not going into details on this as it is not my place to share, I will say my mother and I had a confrontation that left me mildly traumatized and led to me changing a lot of my bad habits when it came to interacting with others.

Now, I lost four years of my college career, and we just covered the first two years I lost. Year one being my mishandling of my math credit, and the second to the battery of surgeries (well, it was technically only half a year I lost, but I lost three semesters to the math debacle, so we still end up with two years). What happened to the fourth year will have a whole chapter dedicated to it, so that only leaves us with what happened to the third year.

But before that, I feel that I need to redress a minor oversight here. I have talked a lot about my back, my heart, my neurological issues, and my height. What I haven't brought up was my eyesight. Firstly, because it was never extremely relevant until now, but also because it did not really occur to me to even talk about it. Having bad eyesight and needing glasses is a mundane and common thing, and plenty of people with absolutely none of my other issues deal with this one. Considering I was about to go into surgery for them, it is now quite relevant to my story.

The funny thing is that I do not remember the world being particularly blurry before I got my first pair of glasses at an early age, and yet I remember all the adults around me being shocked at all the things I could not make out. My parents and nannies would point out things that they felt I should be able to see, only for me to tell them it was too far away to see. That is how I remember it feeling like back then; that all those things were just too far off. It was not until I finally started wearing glasses that I had the proper context for how blurry my vision actually was. So, while I intellectually know that the world really was that blurry back then, that is not how my memory paints it.

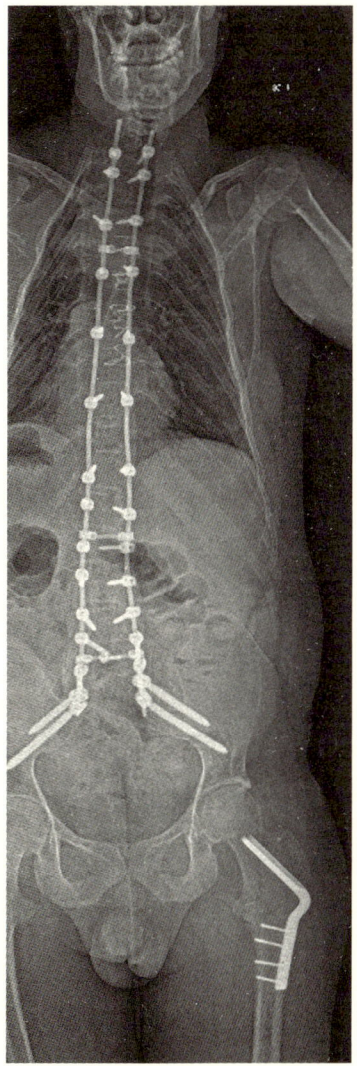
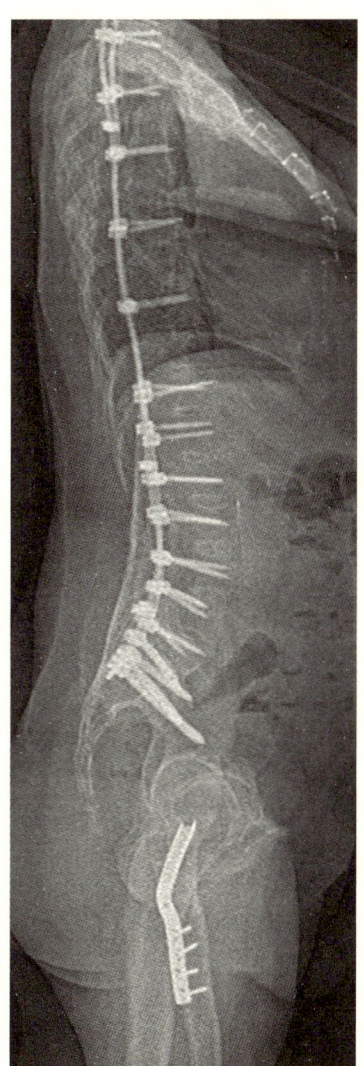

Rods x-ray front view   *Rods x-ray side view*

Now, you may have picked up on "everything looked too far off." Well, that is because I was severely near-sighted. Taking my glasses off created a strange magnifying glass effect immediately in front of my eyes. Enough so that whenever I used a handheld electronic device like a Game Boy (or other portable gaming device) and smart phones, as well as when I read anything (such as books or magazines), I would put whatever it was right in front of my right eye. After taking my glasses off, of course.

You might have caught that bit about my right eye. That because my left eye was far worse than my right. Whenever I read anything, my left eye would drift off so as to allow my right eye to focus, creating a lazy eye effect whenever I read anything, or oddly enough whenever I looked into a mirror. Which leads into the reason for my next batch of surgeries.

What happened was that I went blind in my left eye. Well, no, it never truly went blind, but it got so blurry (even when I was wearing my prescription specs) that it might as well have been. My right eye was not doing that much better, all things being equal. The point being that my eyesight was starting to desert me. You will find that detached lenses, and thus severe nearsightedness, are a very common side effect in those with Marfan syndrome.

This resulted in me getting three eye surgeries, one right after the other, with only a few weeks of recovery in between. Considering how I described my state post-surgery for all the other surgeries that probably sounds horrible. However, eye surgeries left you in a very different state. I only needed to stay one night at the hospital, and I was good to fly back home the day after that. Yes, that involved a lot of flying, but frankly if we had the option, we'd rather be home in Arizona for the winter instead of Baltimore.

This reminds me that the surgeries all took place during the winter of 2013, all of them performed by one Dr. Shine. Also, to be fair, it was only supposed to be two surgeries instead of three. The issue was that during my first surgery, they had me use certain eye drops that ended up causing the new artificial lens to drift upwards into my cornea, resulting in me getting fisheye. The second surgery was them correcting this. They removed that eye drop from my recovery for those last two surgeries.

Now, considering all I just said, you are likely wondering how this lost me a whole year. After all, wasn't this all done over the course of a maybe two months? Well, you would be right, if not for one small little detail: the surgeries rendered me functionally blind for most of the year. I say functionally because my eyes could technically see. The issue was that opening my eyes was so unbelievably painful without preparation (that being special eye drops and medical sunglasses) that I might as well have been blind.

You know all those blind martial arts masters in the movies who can "see" their opponents via sounds? I never quite got to that level, but my other senses were dramatically boosted. Yes, it was that dramatic. I was able to navigate my house via touch, memory, and a cane. More impressive though? My friend Tommy came to Arizona to keep me company as I recovered. It was so good to have him there. I think he may have felt worse than me:

> I can tell you man, it made me feel like multiple contradictory things, because you were the first person I saw in that sorta major condition asides from like, my family, so it was very weird to see that, especially from someone much younger than my parents so it was a really weird… kind of made me realize that young people can suffer through that sort of thing as well. It also kinda made me appreciate life just that little bit more because of it. (Tommy Fisher)

I asked him about being with me after my eye surgery as well:

> The way I felt like when you were going through that process… let's rewind a bit here, I've always known you had issues with seeing in general, and you've already been through a lot of surgeries to begin with! So, it's funny how I viewed it, that he's been through enough surgeries that it's no longer suffering to you, it's just a necessity! At the same time, it was interesting to see you go from pretty much being kinda blind to fully blind. It was interesting to watch you struggle because all the struggles I've seen you go through and just conquer, the one with you having to go blind for a while really was the most interesting one, because you're blind and you're dealing with every other surgery that you've dealt with in your life! You kinda just shoved it off as "Ah! This is just another day in my life! I'll get through this!" I've never seen someone not only just be accepting of what he or she or whatever you want to identify as just take it as a day by day thing, but doesn't complain… by complaining, I mean the whole "oh, woe is me, my life sucks!" Sorta thing! (Tommy Fisher)

This really blew me away. It is nice to have a friend who sees me for who I am and feels some of my pain.

The two of us were both big fans of *Power Rangers* and shows like it, even if my own interest was a touch more ironic than his. Do not get me wrong, several shows in that genre were genuinely good, but so much of it was hilariously cheesy and outright bad, and even the good stuff had its share of camp. Well, Tommy and I decided to binge a particularly cheesy example called *VR Troopers,* a hilariously confused little show that was the result of Saban Entertainment slapping together stock footage of three different shows into one Frankenstein of a product.

My eyes were sealed shut for most of this binging, and yet I have vivid and visual, I repeat visual, memories of it all. My boosted ability to extrapolate information from sound, combined with the few times I could force my eyes open, and I felt like I had actually watched the show instead of just listened to it. Let us just say that I will never underestimate the blind after that.

With all this now completed, I still moved forward within *Christopia* albeit a bit agitated and moved into University at last!

CHAPTER EIGHT:
NEVER-ENDING CHANGES

Giraffe and Hyena watched, flabbergasted, and baffled, at the sight before them. Their fair-weather herd of wildebeest and meerkats and zebras and other such scavengers and prey animals, they were about to get into a turf war with the local rhino herd over control of the watering hole. Frankly, neither group should have had such command over what was supposed to be public space open to all animals. This "herd" of theirs was made to legitimize their part-time control over the area, but the whole sham was finally starting to fall apart before Giraffe's horrified eyes, as he stared on in abject astonishment as the tiny she-monkey got all up in the rhino leader's face, ready to tussle.

The sight of it would have been comical if it was not an omen of such disaster. Of course, Giraffe still possessed some delusions of this ramshackle "herd" of his being a true, long-term ordeal, even if he barely talked to any of them outside of the times they reassumed their occupation of the watering hole. Hyena possessed no such illusions, not any longer; he had found the few worthy of his long-term companionship already and realized the transient nature of all the other relationships quite early. So, he laughed at it all like the Hyena he was.

Right when Giraffe thought teeth and claws were about to get involved, he called the wise elephants to arbitrate before anyone got hurt. The elephants, in all their wisdom, decided that this sham of a herd needed to be disbanded, that the lion pride needed to back off, and that the watering hole was once and forevermore public property to never again be claimed (part time or not) by any one group.

Now, to explain who everyone was in that frankly quite tortured metaphor because that took up a page and I am not repeating myself by just retelling the story sans the animals. We all know who the giraffe was. The hyena was my friend Robert, who has already shared his thoughts with you earlier on, and who I should note did not actually laugh like a hyena in real life when this all went down. I could simply tell that he had found the whole thing darkly amusing. The watering hole was the lounge that the Gaming Club claimed de facto ownership over (and part time de jure ownership). The lion pride was the SCC football team. Let me repeat that, the football team. Us, a bunch of nerds (the only one with combat training being me, and Marfan syndrome made that a very risky position indeed) nearly had a turf war with the football team, with a 5 foot 110 lbs. soaking wet tomboy (our she-monkey) leading the charge. Against the 300 lbs. of muscle that was their leader, with the rest of his team being in that same ballpark. The elephants were the security guards I called in when I feared the fisticuffs were about to happen.

To give a smidgen more context, the football team, annoyed at the Gaming Club's hostile takeover and occupation of the lounge area, decided to push in. They would start using the at the time public televisions to play long, deliberately extended sessions of *Madden* (a football video game; apropos, I know). These would always extend into the beginning of our club meeting times, and they would always plead that we wait for "just one more game to finish!" Eventually we caught on to their game, and that is when the fireworks began.

And that is how the Scottsdale Community College Electronic Gaming Club came to a nearly violent end. Frankly, in retrospect, I am kind of glad that these loons are no longer in my life.

With that out of the way, it is now time to return to and talk about the hiccup in my academic career which centers on my math credit when going for my associates degree at SCC. I devoted some time to that subject earlier on. However, it needs to be addressed as one of the academic dilemmas that kept me at college for far longer than I had hoped for.

I put off doing the long string of required math classes that I needed to complete before being able to take the math course I needed to graduate and move on to university. I did my famous Chris thing of avoiding and delaying until there was literally nothing else needed for my associate's degree left to take. Thus, I ended up stuck for about two years taking one class per semester, artificially lengthening my time in SCC.

Finally, though, I managed to grab that final credit course, and so after an annoying delay, I was ready to graduate from Scottsdale Community College with my associate's degree.

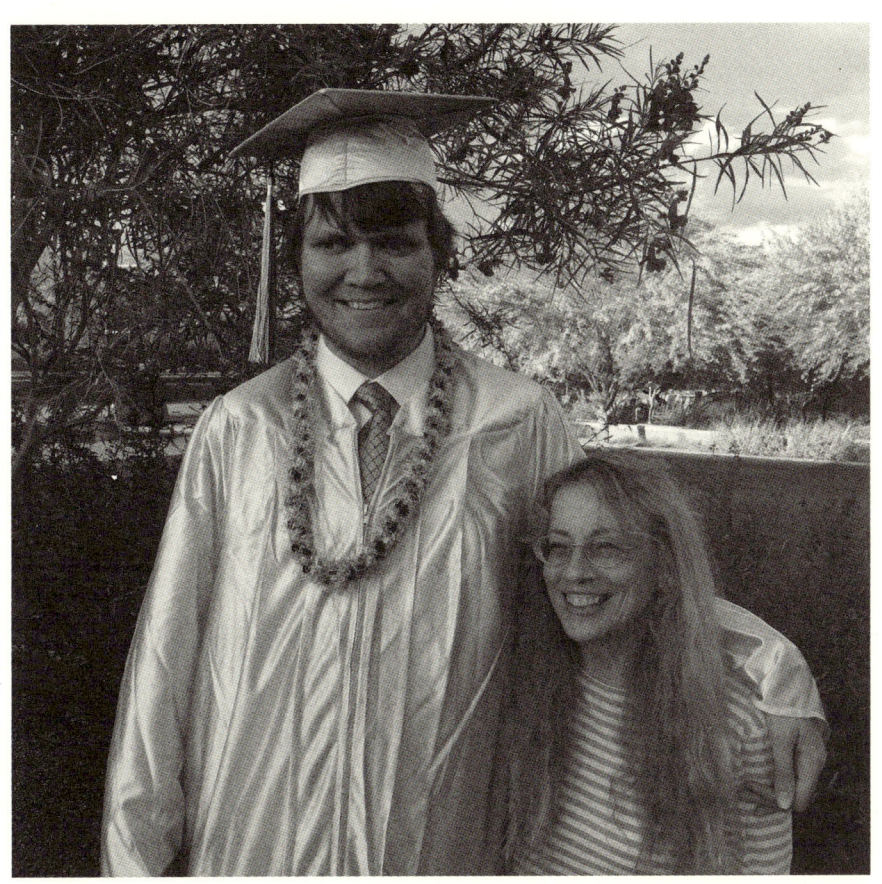

Standing with my long time tutor (and now editor) Patty Tusay on graduation day from Scottsdale Community College

Graduation from SCC at last. Unfortunately, my memory of the event is not the best, for reasons that I will touch upon soon. Of course, this too is another typical Chris thing.

I remember having some difficulty finding my cap and gown. I remember finding the thing to be something of an eyesore. It was blinding bright yellow, bordering on gold in its "luster"; a bit gaudy is what I'm trying to say. Of course, this was all deliberate upon SCC's part. The school colors were the result of a prank the student body played upon the administration back in the 1970s that the school went on to make their own. The administration and student government back then were butting heads over where to prioritize funding. There was a lot of voting and the school colors selected were bright yellow, muddy brown, and puke green. The chosen mascot was the fighting artichoke. The brown was dropped, and the puke green slowly became just green, but the bright yellow and the artichoke? That stayed.

So, there I was, in a bright yellow gown that everyone but I was entranced with. The reason for that disparity in enthusiasm for the thing is closely tied to the reason my memory of the event was so hazy. My fellow students and I and all our various families/friends and fans piled into the large school gymnasium turned theater. Mind you, I had never had cause to go in there before this point. I was not studying dance or theater after all, and I was certainly not a gymnast. I could not even take gym. My parents, my sister, and my tutor Patty Tusay were all there to cheer me on.

I sat down and waited for my turn to get my diploma. As I waited, I got to hear all these speeches from various students who earned certain honors. I got to talk to fellow graduates before and after the ceremony which was kind of nice; I guess I belonged there.

The biggest difference between myself and all those other enthusiastic young minds that night was that, for most of them, this was graduation. Their schooling was done for good, and it was time to go out into the world and make their fortune.

As for myself, I was heading right off to ASU the very next year in pursuit of my major. Therefore, for me, this all felt very fake, like a middle school graduation—a consolation prize on a piece of official paper. Of course, it was not. That associate's degree that the professor in the renaissance hat gave me was a real graduation that happened, it just didn't feel all that real to me due to how quickly I jumped back into the exact same grind I was in before, more school.

This made me feel a bit guilty, warranted or not. Here were all these happy young people celebrating their actual graduation and about to jump into a larger world, and here was grumpy old me feeling like I was given a pat on the head. Yet, despite all this seemingly negative talk, I do not recall being particularly sad during the proceedings. In fact, I remember enjoying the festiveness of it all, the pageantry, and I remember enjoying the fact that everyone else there was enjoying themselves. I knew my friends and family were genuinely happy for me, as there were doubts I would ever make it here. I knew all the other graduates were ecstatic for all the reasons I touched upon earlier. Thus, through all their happiness, I was happy with the proceedings. I think this really may be the first time I felt part of a greater experience and not just into myself. Maybe *Christopia* cannot live forever in a vacuum and the neutral giraffe felt important even if it was short lived.

Sadly, it just did not stick with me the way I know it did with everyone else. It certainly was by no means a bad memory for me, but neither was it a cherished one as I know it likely was for so many others. I guess you can say all that negativity from earlier on with math and general delays from physical issues contributed to my sense of guilt and stymied any long-lasting congratulations.

It was just another manifestation of spinning my wheels in place that I discussed earlier on. But with that, we close the book on Scottsdale Community College, and open the book on Arizona State University and it barely felt all that different.

Oh, there were certainly differences to be had. My assignments were on average more difficult, due dates stricter. There were a lot less tests, with final projects being more in favor than final exams. Though this was likely a result of another difference. I was now pursuing a major and not going after a general education degree. My classes were a lot more focused, and it seems the English department at ASU was not all that enamored with tests.

So yes, things were different. They simply were not fundamentally different, at least not to me. After all, I took no sabbatical after high school. I did not stop to work for a few years either. Next, there I was, going right back to school the very next semester at ASU. However, I can honestly say that my high school graduation did not give me the same feeling. High school feels fundamentally different than college. University does not feel fundamentally different from junior college even though some aspects are different. Some things were the same but not quite, for instance, how I was perceived and now treated by Peter, my stepdad, who had a big hand in my education:

> Well, really, I just figured that by the time you were in college, you were able to handle it. We also knew that Patty was there, you know, so if you had questions on those academic subjects, she would definitely be more adept at handling that then I would be. I mean, while I certainly helped you with math and writing and stuff when you were a kid and a teen, by the time you got to college, all those courses you were doing, even if I had done it back in my day, I had forgotten all of it!

So other than maybe encouraging you; sometimes, you let things slide to the last minute, so I would certainly encourage you to not wait too long to finish homework or do a paper. But that's kind of something that I have always done with you, no matter what school you were in. In terms of telling you what you might want to do, what courses to choose, not my choice. Certainly, by the time you got to ASU, you were capable of doing all that on your own. (Peter Talbert)

There was one other difference though, and that is, I had no consistent on-campus friend group like I did at SCC. I think my generally negative experiences with the Electronic Gaming Club, plus the more politically charged nature of university student bodies, resulted in my deciding against going through that all over again lest I get involved in a gang war between the theater kids and the STEM field students or something. Therefore, I was going it alone except for my one-on-one peer mentor and occasional sightings of my old high school peer, Lee, and off-campus friend, Robert. And that will be it for school for the time being. Obviously, it was still happening, but for the most part, it was the same old grind as it always was, aside from the minute differences I already covered. Obviously, things happened, but not really in a way that is relevant to the subject of this book. I had other things going on in my life.

It is time to introduce another player in the stage production known as my life; Barbara Sause and only now, after having typed that name upon this page, do I realize how much it sounds like "Barbecue Sauce." My second roommate, and part of the impetus for moving out of our apartment and into the house I currently co-own and live within.

I do not know her story quite as well as I know Liz's, but I will give some quick basics. She is Liz's best friend, though unlike my mother, they met each other sometime later in life. She is very, very into horses (and this plays a big role in certain elements of the house we end up moving into) and used to work with them professionally (and still works with them as a passion hobby) in New Jersey. That is, until Hurricane Sandy hit. That's when Liz first offered to let her move in, and while she would stay at the apartment for increasingly long stretches, she did not permanently move in with us, and to the sunny state of Arizona in general, until we moved into the house permanently. Considering what she ultimately ended up using our large backyard for, the reason for the wait was obvious to me, horses. Barbara likes to tell the story in her own words:

> I worked with horses, and so that means I work outside all winter. That is a big advantage for Arizona. Then Hurricane Sandy hit... during which we lost power, were surrounded by snow, and during it all I'm

wondering "what am I doing here? I should move to Arizona!" So, I put my notice in and here I am! You guys [myself and Liz] were happy here, so I thought "let's give this a try!" Oh right, almost forgot, it was only AFTER you got this house that I seriously thought to move permanently. As you remember, before I would only come to visit. The old place was too small for me, and Liz was always at work, so I would just drive around the area and I saw this neighborhood. I told Liz if we could buy a place here with a casita or something. Liz mentions this to your mom, she thought it was a great idea. Few years later, there was a "For Sale" sign! So, once you guys bought this, with room for horses, I love horses, so I had my impetus to move out here! (Barbara Sause)

I will have been living in the new house going on five years. At first sight, the place seemed too good to be true. Almost purposely built to keep me here in Arizona, back in a time where I was thinking about scrounging up funds to move to either Seattle or back to New York City. Chicago also came up, as my biological dad lived there, but Seattle and New York got the most consideration. I would later learn of a number of factors that blew this out of the water as the sole reason this happened, such as the fact that Liz had already been eyeing the place and she was building up funds for a while, what Barbara would end up converting the lawn into, etc.:

Well, to turn the clock back to give a bit of context, I will start with meeting Barb at a Bible study type thing... prayer meeting, Bible study, that type of thing... And, uh... Well, it was during a very bad period of my life when one of my best friends died from cancer... So [Barbara] helped me quite a bit in that grieving process, so we became best friends... And of course, I was still best friends with your mom too! Three amigos! So just having two of my most dear friends here in Arizona, being here with them, that was amazing, but while I was always happy whenever Barbara would come over to visit, when she did drive around and said to me, 'I would love to move out here full time, if we could just get one of these larger places...' Well, I was just thrilled at the idea! Basically, that is it! After Barb suggested it, your mom and I did everything we could to make it happen! (Liz Foldi)

I still cannot help but have my suspicions that trying to keep me from moving out of state was not at least part of the reason my parents decided to help Liz buy that home.

It was a large property in a ranching neighborhood. I already know that is probably conjuring images of the huge ranches like Skywalker Ranch, that we owned the entire hillside and that our nearest neighbors were two miles away, but no. This was an actual neighborhood, with houses visibly next to the other like in any other neighborhood. What made it a ranching neighborhood was that everyone had a huge backyard and were legally allowed to keep and raise livestock and horses upon these plots of land, and many of those living in this neighborhood did. There's a donkey I call Dunkey (I have no idea what his real name is; don't know his owner, and I never felt the need to rectify that) that I like to pet whenever I take my mile-long walks through the neighborhood, and there are a lot of horses and chickens about upon that same route.

The house itself is large. Four bedrooms (one reserved as a guest bedroom, three in use), four bathrooms, large garage, a combination kitchen/dining area, a living room, and a storage area that we converted into a second living room for my own personal use. While the place is still a very nice-looking place even today, the way the old owners had everything set up gave the place a one-story manor feel to it; to the point that it's price tag, which in retrospect was a bit high for a single story property, seemed like a too-good-to-be-true steal. Part of that was of course do to the former occupants bringing out the nines and cleaning everything to a shine that could be seen from space. Yet the simple fact was that the stuff they had seemed a lot more expensive than what we ultimately ended up replacing it all with when we moved in and they moved out (and we weren't trying to be frugal or anything). Ostentatious king-sized beds, pricey gym equipment. Frankly I swear, I remember spotting a sports car in the driveway when we came to inspect the property; the former owner seemed to be the right age to be having a mid-life crisis, and what we saw screamed it.

Yet, all of that is said in retrospect. At the time, when I was first bucking at the mostly nonexistent chains my parents had upon me, it really did look like a bribe to not leave the state as I had been discussing at the time. Most of these chains were placed there by myself when I decided to focus upon school, to not work, and thus to become financially reliant upon my parents. After being forcibly stuck in the academic grind longer than I should have, even these fake chains started to chafe, and I was starting to gain some of my inheritance from my grandfather at the time that I suggested I would use to move. Only to have this (from my perspective at that time) too-perfect property dropped in my lap. I even said as much when I went out to sushi with my parents to celebrate the purchase of the place. It was then that both mom and Liz revealed to me that the latter had already been eyeing up such a property since Barbara expressed interest in moving in with us, and frankly I was quite chagrined at myself at the conclusion of that conversation. The universe does not revolve around me after all.

Why would Barbara moving in require such a large property in the first place? Remember how I said Miss Sause has a passion for equines? And how we were legally allowed to keep horses and other livestock upon these properties? Barbara ended up buying three horses after converting the old backyard into a proper pasture. One chestnut named Sophia, one Arabian named Alouda, and one miniature named Adea.

In short, it was a convincing case that, at least with most parties involved, this was not some long con to keep me and my hundred and one medical maladies in this state and in sight. Though I suspect mom was nonetheless relieved when I did indeed decide to stay in the state for the time being for that very reason. However, we all loved the house. My roommates were worried that some of my behaviors would become problematic. You see, living in *Christopia* one did not really think of others first:

> I have seen, since we have been living together, I have seen such a difference in you, Chris. Such growth! You used to come in and not be aware of anyone's feelings... stuff like coming out to the kitchen at two in the morning and being loud, not caring about the noise. After I complained, you went from that to coming in at two in the morning and being quiet! Because you would be aware that people were sleeping. For you, that was such a huge thing! (Barbara Sause)

Liz and Barbara began discussing more changes I made since we moved into the house:

> Just to be aware of your roommates is fantastic! Now we have gotten to the point that we go to bed early because we get up early, but you have organized your evening to be done in the kitchen by 9 PM. So, you are totally considerate of your roommates! I think God set this up to help you become considerate of people! When we have guests, you come out and introduce yourself, during the holidays you are considerate of friends and family. When I met you, you weren't like that at all. I think having roommates has helped you, and it's helped us. It has really been perfect! (Barbara Sause)

Liz chimed in with:

> Yeah, I agree completely with Barbara and what she just said. I also see that change. The maturity. I mean, you have just grown, and we have grown, and it has been a good experience for all of us because

we all have to learn to be considerate. I have learned things myself. But the wonderful thing is that there is a communal feeling. You have roommates, but it is not just like roommates, it is like a family! That is what feels good, and that is how I see it. (Liz Foldi)

Considering what was to come next, my mother's worries were not just empty paranoia.

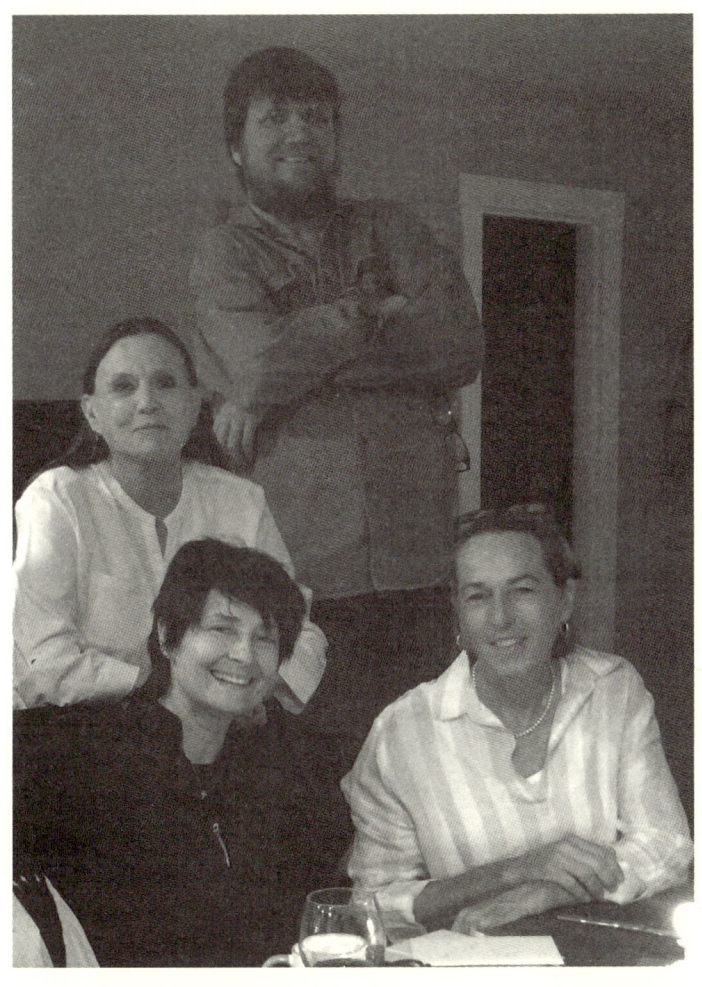

With my Mom and housemates Liz Foldi and Barbara

CHAPTER NINE:
PISSING OFF THE GIRAFFE

What I am about to write about, as the chapter title may suggest (as well as the last lines of the last chapter), is frankly one of the hardest moments of my life. At least, from my personal perspective, perhaps from my parent's and loved one's perspective, my first heart operation or my spinal surgeries were more harrowing, and I was just too oblivious to care. However, considering that those were planned out far in advanced, and were known situations in a way that this was not, not even mentioning my own misery during the whole ordeal, let us say I doubt that my loved ones and I see things all that differently in this regard.

This all happened during the year of 2016, that is, the vast bulk of what I wish to touch upon in this segment. There is a certain irony to all this, I suppose; that year had gained a reputation, bordering on running joke in the collective unconscious, of being the worst year in modern human history. One well-known talk show host, comedian John Oliver, made a huge show of "blowing up" 2016 at the conclusion of the year to show his disgust for that span of 366 days (it was a leap year). I believe that reputation to be heavily exaggerated when it comes to humanity, most of it fueled by the election not going the way anyone thought it would and the resultant hysteria around that. However, for me, it really was the worst year in history.

I cannot recall the exact date of the instigating incident, the moment this year-long trek through my personal hell began, because at the time, I had dismissed it as a particularly painful but ultimately unimportant night of my twenty-six-year-old life. Something to tell stories about with friends, family, maybe my kids and grandkids someday about how much heartburn and food poisoning can suck, particularly if you have Marfan syndrome, but ultimately not pivotal enough to mark the date. How wrong I was, I know, but it would be a few months until I knew exactly what had happened that night. I will say that it was late winter though, perhaps early spring.

John Greer, my martial arts instructor, and I had a bit of a tradition. I was his personal protégé at this time; he had lost his formal school to a lot of things that were going on. However, he still retained enough authority to advance us in belt ranks. After I had reached some milestone or if he just wanted to hang out as he was also my best friend, he would take me to a restaurant or other food establishment of my choice. The one restriction is that it had to be something within his price range, so going out for sushi was the priciest we ever got. No expensive steak dinners or lobsters for us. We often brought other friends along.

What this usually translated into was some manner of fast-food joint or salad bar. One place I had become particularly fond of back then was a franchise known as Five Guys Burgers and Fries. Five Guys is known to have the tastiest burgers by fast-food standards, as they simply did not adhere to a lot of the restrictions that the more mainstream establishments were mired in. They cooked things in fatty bacon grease and peanut oil, and they were proud of it. While that made for incredibly tasty food, it also made for less than heathy food. A heart attack in a bun fits this meal. This is the primary reason we did not rush immediately to the hospital when I started feeling the most intense chest, back, and stomach pain of my life. We thought we were dealing with a combination of severe heartburn, food poisoning, and indigestion, and we had a former Marine medic's stamp of approval on that theory. Now, there is reasonable chance I still would have gone to the hospital regardless and would have had those illusions dashed far earlier than they were, except that I was in such agony that a car trip to the emergency room followed by waiting in the waiting room sounded intolerable. John said he knew how to soothe my pain now, while I stayed in bed in my room at my parents' place, and by God, he did just that. He made that agonizing night tolerable and helped me make a full recovery the next day.

Of course, it was not heartburn, food poisoning, nor indigestion, of any severity. It was my descending aorta dissecting, and from that day forward, I was rolling the dice on whether I survived to see the morning or not, and had zero idea my life was constantly on a knife's edge. It was rather terrifying when, years later, I did research, and saw exactly what my odds of survival had been every day from the dissection to when I finally got my operation. They were quite low. My purpose here is to inform and educate, not needlessly scare people, and frankly the fact that those odds got so low was on me. What I will say is that if you or your loved ones with Marfan syndrome, or just someone you suspect may have the affliction, ever feel these combinations of symptoms, you may wish to check into the emergency room instead of gambling the way I unintentionally did.

I really should have been clued in that something was up earlier than I was, before my doctors at Johns Hopkins had to spell it out flat out for me. Several weird and bizarre issues began to sprout up here and there. Strange bouts of breathlessness, unexplained chest pains, etc. I remember getting sicker easier than I usually did, though my immune system is not exactly the greatest at the best of times, so this one could be pure coincidence and I just caught a few more bugs than usual. The strangest and worst of these odd occurrences was a severe limp in my right leg along with accompanying leg pains that came and went. I went to visit Tommy in New York for a week, and my leg started acting up there as well. I remember one time we walked from his place to a restaurant with no difficulty, only for me to call an Uber to take us back after dinner because my leg started to act up. The driver sent me a confused text when he saw how short of a distance we were traveling, but seemed to quickly understand what was up when he saw me walk out of Naruto Ramen with a very noticeable limp and hanging off my friend's very broad shoulders. Tommy asked if I wanted to see a doctor, but like hell did I want to interrupt my time with him by risking hospitalization; I would rather just muscle through it like I did most things. I did not say it like that of course. I simply said that I had already dealt with this before and was in no danger, and I could handle this, deliberately leaving vague what "dealt with this before" implied. I was not going to outright lie to my best friend, akin to a brother really, over this, but if he interpreted that as Chris had already seen the doctor and had done all he could, then I was not going to stop him from thinking that. What I really meant when I said had dealt with it before was that I had managed to just tough it out and endure it before, and that I was confident in my ability to do so again.

Honestly, that is the crux of this issue, why did I not seek medical advice when I really should have when these issues keep cropping up. I only came to realize that what I experienced was more than a one-time food related debacle when I went for my annual at Johns Hopkins, and that would be my primary coping mechanism. One of my greatest strengths, but also a potentially fatal weakness in this case, was the extreme pain tolerance I had grown, along with, more importantly, the attitude of just enduring the tough times and focusing on enjoying myself as much as I could. I have certainly been praised on this matter; my ability to just live life despite all the physical difficulties—more concerned with keeping up-to-date with nerd culture and the Internet than with complaining—has gained me much admiration, and I consider this trait more than a mere net positive in my life. I would be a very miserable person, maybe flat out insane or suicidal, if not for this. Be that as it may, it also results in my deciding to simply tough things out when I really should seek help. It's not even as a matter of pride or strength either; I simply do not want to be inconvenienced and pulled away from my nerdy pursuits, and, say, going to see the doctor would certainly do that. One particularly extreme example of this; one time, I am pretty sure I nearly had a heart attack. Once that was over, I knew I really should have called an ambulance, but ultimately, I decided not to because I wanted to sleep instead. I knew that was a dumb decision when I woke up the next day, but still decided that it had passed and just went on with my life (though I did swear to myself that if I ever felt anything like that again, I would immediately call 911. Luckily, I have never had to).

Though to be a bit fair to myself, I had no real way of knowing that the limp and the Five Guys incident were at all related back then, nor do I know for certain that they were connected at all as this is all ad hoc guesswork. Confident guesswork that I would bet good money upon, but ad hoc guesswork all the same, not that it was relevant by the time we did learn what was happening. Whether I could connect those two dots or not doesn't really change the fact that when things got as bad as they did when I was visiting Tommy that the intelligent thing would have been to check into an ER to see what exactly was wrong.

And so, life went on for me, oblivious to the ticking time-bomb my heart had become the entire time. Winter came to an end, spring came and went, I finished a semester of school and then my tutors and I set up my classes for next semester, and why wouldn't I? I had no reason to believe I would be unable to attend. After all that was done, came summer vacation. I enjoyed a few weeks of complete freedom, before my parents and I packed up and flew off to Baltimore, usually for unpleasant reasons for my annual checkup in June. We were going to be there for four days, before flying back to Arizona to enjoy the rest of my summer vacation before resuming school come September. We even had plans to meet mom's side of the family in Washington State, as we tend to do every year in some manner. This was all so utterly routine, is what I am trying to get at. Once there, I went through the usual battery of echocardiograms and x-rays and CAT scans. After an odious and tedious day of this (maybe two days, cannot quite recall), my parents and I waited to discuss the results in Dr. Hal Dietz's office.

When Dr. Dietz arrived with a grim look on his face, he told us flat out that my descending aorta had dissected, and that I would be dead by Christmas if I did not go in for surgery as soon as possible. We had expected to be staying in Baltimore for the usual routine four days. We ended up being stuck there for four months. I think I will let Peter start to tell some of this from the traumatic family perspective.

> When we flew to Baltimore with Chris for his annual checkup in early June, we presumed we would be staying for 3 days. The moment we discovered that he had an aortic dissection, we realized that we would be there considerably longer. We could not have imagined that we would be there until mid-September. Once he'd been admitted, we checked out of the Four Seasons hotel and booked an extended stay reservation at the

> local Marriott Residence Inn on Light St. We had long since given up on staying at the Harbor Court hotel as Chris had terrible and painful memories from staying there for months after his back operation. Going to their small gym every morning around 5 am, I would see the same people for a week or two and then they'd be gone, replaced by a new fitness fanatic who'd be there for another week or two and then, poof, be gone as well. There was always a mini competition to see who could arrive first to get the treadmill and not the stationary bike. (Peter Talbert)

Hearing this from my dad while conducting these interviews also made me feel guilty, because I really did not have horrible memories of the place. I only had horrible memories of the pain, but I did not associate that pain with the location. If my parents had wished to stay at the Harbor Hotel, I would have been chill with that. Peter continues:

> We became experts at Uber, having rarely used them previously. Like clockwork, Uber to JH at 9 am, then back to our home (the Marriott started to feel like home after a month) at 5 pm. A full workday. Lunches at the JH cafeteria were another ritual, looked forward to greatly to break up the monotony of PPE gowns, gloves, and masks (who knew the routine would presage COVID-19 by several years) while sitting in the unforgiving hospital chairs next to Chris's bed. Annie was mostly salads and sandwiches and I was veggie wraps and sushi when available. At night, back at the hotel/home, Annie had discovered the joys of Stouffer's meat loaf which they sold next to the front desk in a small refrigerator. (Peter Talbert)

All I knew was that the surgery was not scheduled to happen for another two days after that fateful diagnosis. Looking back, I am quite glad I did not know the sort of odds I had been dealing with that whole time, or I would have immediately demanded I get rushed into surgery right then and there. Frankly, I am a bit surprised that my doctors had not insisted on doing just that. However, I am glad I did have those last two days to reflect and inform everyone of what just happened. It also gave me enough time to withdraw from the next semester and give ASU the necessary medical records to explain why I would not be attending until next year. It gave me time to come to terms with all of this, so I was not a nervous wreck when the time came.

It also allowed me time to come to a somewhat startling realization; I was freaking angry. I never got angry about this sort of thing, I never let myself get angry about this sort of thing. This sort of thing was to be expected and accepted, lest I become a sad shell of a man I have seen others become when they had to deal with my sort of severe circumstances. This giraffe, who for so long was completely neutral to the realities of his own existence, began to truly envy, and maybe resent, the water buffalo, gazelle, and lions. Because they were water buffalo, gazelle, and lions, and did not have to deal with all the misery that came from being a giraffe and that just was not fair. It just was not fair at all. Could it be *Christopia* was unraveling right before my eyes?

What was so different between now and the rest of my life up to that point, was that this would happen now. I mean, this is obviously not the first time I have let my less-than-ideal circumstances get to me to some degree as circumstances suck, and I'm only human. Stuff like not being able to properly compete in the martial arts, and a bevy of other things brought on by the no contact sports and the constantly watch your heart rate like a hawk rule. However, that would always only last if I were dealing with that situation and quickly fade to the back of my mind when said situation ceased to be my focus. This felt bone deep, this contempt and anger, the sort I have seen wither others away when I was staying in the hospital those times I had to come in for surgery. While I have exorcised these deep negative emotions from myself and have regained what I would consider normal homogeneity, since that day, I have had moments when I am alone where I just hate all this misery that's been dumped upon me in a way I just never did before.

Back to the question of what exactly, if anything, was different to cause all this angst? Honestly, it is the fact that this was completely unplanned. This was the first time Marfan syndrome completely flipped my life upside down out of nowhere. Everything else was planned. I knew ahead of time that I would be out of the game during certain months, and why. Oh, unexpected things certainly happened. No one was prepared for just how disabling (frankly, flat out crippling) my spinal surgery would be or how long I would need to recover; no one was planning to need to take me home in an RV, and I certainly wasn't expecting to still be in fairly severe pain even when I started school again. Yet, that was all adjustments made to a plan we already had. This hit me out of nowhere like an eighteen-wheeler at midnight while I listened to an iPod full of heavy metal songs with my eyes closed.

The day came, my surgery to be done by Dr. Black. Yes, I know, it sounds like I just stepped into a medical drama with a name like that. His father must have murdered ten men, including the father of his lovely nurse, and he became a doctor to save score more lives than that to atone for the sins of the father. Or he killed those ten men and became a doctor because he found saving lives to be more satisfying than murder. Or he is secretly a superhero that hunts demons. I still had the ability, even in this dreadful situation, to make up scenarios as if I were that child of long ago headed in for his first surgery. Maybe all was not lost.

While I never remember passing out, I remember a bit more than I usually would. For one, I rarely remember talking to my doctors as they set up the surgery room, though I'm fairly sure that was because they applied the anesthesia later than usual this time. I remember talking about how absurd the final arc of the Naruto anime was shaping up to be (oh how naïve I was back then, not realizing this "final arc" would be dragged out so much as to account for a third of the entire series). I then remember waking up and feeling like I was ripped to shreds and was just barely patched back together. When I saw all of me, I realized that was pretty much the case; I was covered in temporary medical implants, strange silver cylinders I could not for the life of me recall the function of were inserted into (and later removed from) my skin like flash drives into USB ports. I had a breathing apparatus inserted into my esophagus that stayed there for longer than the norm for this sort of thing. The scar that indicated where they opened me up for the surgery, it frankly looked like I survived a shark attack. My entire left side was peeled off down to the hip and was then stitched back together. It makes me a bit sick to think about all of this even now. Again, Peter's perspective on my actual surgery is welcome to me as I was unaware of so much my family was going through. Here I was getting angry at myself, and everyone was seeing me as a superhero:

> But the days were mostly about sitting with Chris during the days, getting him water or ice chips when he was allowed, and reading his messages on the whiteboard as he was unable to speak because of the tracheotomy. He found some diversion watching TV, mostly it seemed tuned to Shark Week. There were always nurses wandering in to check on him, and usually once a day Dr. Black, his surgeon, would stop by to see his progress. It was often two steps forward, one step back. He at one point needed to have an IVC (inferior vena cava filter) implanted to prevent a blood clot from traveling to his heart. And occasionally his heart rate would get so elevated that I feared his heart might burst, at one point hitting 163 bpm. His chest was vibrating so hard. I was terrified until they managed to bring it back down. Chris is normally on medication that keeps his heart low, and he's never supposed to exceed 115 bpm. When he was finally able to sit up and leave his bed, at first it was a matter of shuffling two steps to a chair next to the bed. With so many tubes and IVs to account for, just this small expedition took 20 minutes, and was exhausting. Weeks later he started to make walks around the hallways, again with all manner of paraphernalia attached, and me pushing a chair on rollers right behind him so he could sit every few yards when the effort proved too taxing. That day he made it around the entire hallway was a major milestone. Extra meatloaf that night! And through it all, Chris was incredible. He dealt

with every obstacle and setback and just kept persevering. He was beyond amazing—a superhero in every respect. (Peter Talbert)

Wow, it really touches me that they thought I was so amazing! However, physically, and emotionally, so much more was happening with me.

I was incapable of talking and would be effectively mute for months to come. I would not recover my full voice for months after I returned to Arizona. That it recovered on its own and without surgery was something of a miracle, a fact that made my religious roommates quite smug. I was incapable or drinking any liquid substances for months. Though I did sneak the occasional bit of melted water from the ice cubes I was given to deal with my frequent fevers. They feared liquids ingested through the mouth would gather in my lungs.

I was incapable of eating physical food likewise for months. Like what was done for hydration, I also got my nutrition via IV drip. Unlike water, I had no way of sneaking any of the real stuff into me. This bit was not too unusual compared to how long it would be until I would be able to drink.

I dealt with that first hurdle via my phone. That little device never left my side, the access it gave me to the Internet and through that, the wider world was an unbelievable boon to my sanity, though I cannot help but think that it developed into something of an addiction that I still have a hard time throwing off. In fact, I still have issues of unconsciously pulling my phone out at inappropriate times, in a way I really did not before this point. It also allowed me to communicate with my friends and family, who rarely left my side (they took shifts and only left me alone when the hospital forced the issue), by typing out what I wanted to say on my phone. I even got an app that verbalized what I typed out, and we all got a good chuckle from the way it mangled the pronunciation of certain words. I had no issues with hearing, luckily, so no accommodations had to be made for that.

The second hurdle caused me to live vicariously through videos about water and other drinks. I became an expert on water in all its forms, and nearly bought a years' worth of some really pricey spring water because a *YouTube* channel that specialized in reviewing and simply drinking water on camera, of all things, told me that this brand was the best on the planet. While my absolute obsession with H2O would wane when I became reacquainted with other liquids (like soda) months later, I admit I kind of wish I had gone through with that. Lord knows my waistline would sing my praises if I was still a water fanatic like I was immediately upon regaining the ability to drink, instead of falling back on bad old habits of consuming a lot of caffeinated/sugary drinks.

As for that final hurdle concerning food. Well, I got really into watching competitive eaters do their things. Watch them devour an uncomfortable amount of food so that I may live vicariously through them. Through them, I too ate that pile of two hundred hotdogs in ten minutes. I really got to learn what their lives were like; they tend to be healthy eaters with strenuous workout routines when not devouring literal kilos' worth of unhealthy and greasy foods.

And so, it went. I would be there for four months, so frankly if I wanted to (and if I could scrounge up enough memories) I could devote this entire book to just this one experience. Much happened. I would eventually get a tracheostomy tube, for one, and then later had it removed. I finally left the ICU after being there for almost three months, longer than I was stuck in normal recovery. That is not how this thing usually works, and it was kind of freaky to be stuck amongst the often terminally ill for so long, but it made sense. My immune system was not weakened upon the conclusion of my surgery. My immune system had flat out ceased to exist upon the conclusion of my surgery. That is why I had those ice cubes from which I could smuggle liquid water into myself (before they wised up and put it in taped over towels or just gave me ice packs); I had a massive fever that never abated for months. I had the flu, I had pneumonia, I had the common cold, I had a thousand bacterial infections, I had everything short of an uncurable disease like HIV or cancer. I am pretty sure I would have gotten COVID-19 if this had happened today. Once my immune system returned from its trip to Tahiti, having enjoyed the company of the immune systems of some supermodels, I was finally cleared to go to the normal recovery ward. I would start my physical therapy and learn that my ability to breath was permanently gimped; I would get short of breath far, far easier from then on. Soon, the time to leave was upon me.

However, it was delayed three times. This sure made me angry. I punched my desk as I wrote that line, the sheer frustration of being stuck there for even a second longer was so potent. The third time I was told that my time leaving was to be delayed, I snapped. I grabbed the poor intern that had to deliver that news by the collar and demanded to know why they were denying me my freedom. What right did they have to keep me imprisoned for even a minute longer?! She immediately fled. Yes, she was four-foot nothing and I am a seven-foot tree of a man. I was terrified that my burst of anger would come to destroy my reputation, make me some social pariah. Never mind the fact that she was an abled bodied medical student, and I was a barely functional hospital patient who needed a wheelchair to get anywhere. She was a tiny Asian woman, and I was a seven-foot ogre. Luckily, nothing came of it. But the fact that I was so absolutely done with being trapped there, that I let myself get into a situation like that to begin with, tells you something about what I was going through.

Eventually though, they finally let me go. My parents and I stayed in Baltimore for a week or so getting everything squared away before we flew back to Arizona and the rest of my life.

CHAPTER TEN:
GETTING IT TOGETHER

I admit, getting old has become something of a mild source of anxiety for me lately. I already have enough issues right now in my relative youth, so it is a bit nerve-wracking to consider what will come with age. The point, however, stands; I do not have much to worry about going forwards as far as Marfan syndrome is concerned.

    I would like to say that we returned to Arizona with a feeling of relief in our minds, but that would be less than true. Not because we were worried about future incidents, no, there were no anxieties on that front. Rather, we were too busy dealing with the immediate issues that came with my recovery now that I had returned home from the hospital to concern ourselves over more anxiety in the future.

    It is a tad funny to compare my spinal surgery to this latest one. By all rights, the former had a far worse recovery period, the pain was often worse, and the long-term ramifications were far grander. Yet, it was the latter that got the closest to breaking me emotionally. There are a few reasons for this, but one I think is how much of that recovery time involved me confined to the hospital. Yes, I needed a few years to fully recover from the spinal surgery (compared to the second heart surgery taking about half a year's time), but I spent the vast majority of that outside of the hospital and in Arizona, at home. I was only in the hospital for a few weeks, and then in Baltimore for another month after that before road tripping home. I was not trapped in the hospital for four months, and frankly suffering all this at home makes a huge difference. Another huge difference is that I was a good deal younger. I was still 18 after all, and thus I had a lot more energy to devote to enduring this.

I bring this up to point out that upon arriving home from the hospital, I only spent the next few months (and not the next year) returning to personal homeostasis. The biggest issue was my voice. I had luckily recovered the ability to speak, but I had yet to recover my voice. In its place was a raspy whisper, my throat rough-sounding as if I were a life-long chain smoker. Worse news was that, by all rights, I was past the point where I was supposed to recover said voice naturally, and that I would eventually have to fly back to get a bit of minor surgery done to fix it. You can guess what a joy news like that would have been for us at the time. The last time we went in for something minor and routine, I ended up in the ICU for months. Of course, we understood there would not be a repeat of that here, unless by some absurd evil miracle I had somehow developed throat cancer (I did not, by the way). Thus, we were prepared to fly back to Baltimore to get my throat fixed in a month or so.

Then, out of the blue, my voice came back. I was ecstatic, of course, if a bit confused. After all, I was told under no uncertain terms that if it had not returned on its own by that point, that my voice was gone without surgery. Of course, when we told the doctors, they were also surprised, but ultimately told me that this was not totally unprecedented. My roommates, who had been praying for my voice to return, saw this as their prayers being answered. Oh, and when I say praying, I do not use that term lightly with them; this was not the sort of easy bedtime praying we were taught as kids, no quick drop to the knees with hand clasped and a few whispered words. My roommates are devout Christians, and they asked entire choirs at their church to ask God for help. I may not be exactly the religious sort, so I have my personal doubts on the efficacy of their labors, but I was nonetheless grateful and more than willing to let them take the credit for this. Getting my voice back, without having to go under the scalpel one more time, truly was a miracle, after all.

The other part of my recovery was simply getting my stamina back and getting to the point where I was not breathless every time I crossed the room. I must admit, I never quite reached my pre-surgery levels of stamina, a constant reminder of what I had to go through, a metaphorical scar to accompany my literal ones. There are times I will go walking and suddenly feel an overwhelming need to stop and just let my heart rate return to normal, and I am initially just confused. After all, my usual rest point was just right ahead of me, surely, I can last one more minute. Then, I remember why exhaustion, so suddenly and arbitrarily came upon me, and I am reminded of what I have lost and most likely for good. Heck, on the matter of breathlessness, I still occasionally get breathless when I simply cross a room, though very rarely now and usually only because the rest of my day was busy. A sort of buildup, from the day. One thing I have noticed is that I almost always go through about thirty seconds of breathless panting once I lie down again after exerting myself to any degree. The funny thing is that the amount I had exerted myself did not really seem to correlate with how much I had to pant before my breathing returns to normal. Take out the trash, lie down, pant for thirty seconds. Go through the entirety of my black belt forms from front to back, collapse into bed physically exhausted, pant for thirty seconds.

While all of this was quite huge to be sure, I still cannot touch my toes, not since my spinal surgery more than a decade ago now. In the end, as I said last chapter, the biggest difference was that one procedure was planned, the other was a complete surprise.

From that point on, however, life certainly did not stop for me. I had accomplishments, I had failures, and thus stories to tell. Not quite as many as I feel I should. After all, we are discussing a four-year period of history here, between the surgery and now. But frankly, I kind of kept my head down when I hit University, at least when it came to on-campus activities. There seemed to be sudden protests and riots popping off for every little thing at universities all over the world, and frankly, with the way my SCC friend/social group imploded in on itself, I kept a low profile. I had no desire to make waves or even make permanent friends.

That is not to say that my life was completely dull and without radical change; it was not. Trust me, if the me of six years ago were to meet modern me, he would likely be at least initially horrified, though I feel I could debate him to my point of view given time. Fat chance of that happening if I were confronted by my eighteen-year-old self; I would be indistinguishable from the enemy by young and dumb me. But you see, most of that change was a change in life philosophy and political thought, and most of that achieved by being a passive participant in the culture wars. As Liz Foldi and my dad Peter said earlier, I have changed in knowing when to speak about certain things and when not to, especially not just for argument's sake. I was still moving forward in life and at ASU.

My graduation was coming fast. And the story of my graduation, and boy is it quite the story at that, is at hand. It, like many a college milestone story, involved a drug bender but not what you think. This bender of mine was a complete accident and involved no illegal substances. I do, however, suffer from a severe case of ADHD, and I have been medicated for it. The stimulants I use are dang powerful, more so than mere Adderall by that point, and make sleep impossible for a period. Frankly, I believe I have grown something of a reliance on it, and caffeine, when it comes to waking up in the morning. Even if I get a solid nine hours of sleep, without a combination of my Cotempla (the medication I take now; I have rotated through quite a few prescriptions) and either coffee or some manner of caffeinated soda, I will still feel like the living dead. I have luckily been assured by my therapists and doctors that I can indeed ween myself off this easily enough. I would feel like garbage for about a week, but because it is not actually a chemical addiction, I would be fine after that period was up, and back to normal after said period. But for now, I needed to survive in academia and the world and would think about all that at a better time.

I knew my graduation was going to require that I be awake at about seven o'clock in the morning. That is not an hour I have an easy time waking up at. Often, the sheer anxiety of having to get up at that time just keeps me up all night. This has always been a bit of an issue with me, especially as my circadian rhythm got more and more screwed up by a combination of my own horrible habits (video games, Internet addiction and procrastination) and schoolwork. Let me tell it to you straight up: my usual bedtime these days is four in the morning. I am just glad that, as an author, I for the most part make my own schedule, and I'm actually rather good with all-nighters. I can adjust to normal times, but it always comes with at least a few sleepless nights as I toss and turn and then realize I need to be up in a mere two hours and just give up and take advantage of my lack of sleep to fall asleep early the coming night and wake up on demand, fully rested.

And that right there, is the most important rung in the sequence of unfortunate and bizarre events that was my graduation. Let us rewind just a touch, though. After all, I said this was the most important rung on this rickety ladder, not the first one. This was my graduation, and everyone who was anyone in my life was supposed to come, and a huge portion of them did. Some who could not, made me sad but it was understandable; we were not sure if my Uncle Dick and Aunt Jan were even capable of traveling anymore at that point (they certainly cannot now), for example. Two people who should have been coming, the centerpiece if you will, were my biological father, Jim Stuart, and my best friend Tommy Fisher. Unfortunately, both had to back out at the last minute, both for personal medical reasons that made flying at the time of my graduation impossible for them. I even started joking that I expected my graduation ceremony to be ground zero for the zombie apocalypse. Later, I found out that my class was the last graduating class to have a live ceremony thanks to COVID-19, so that joke ended up being morbidly prescient.

But now we return to that main rung. That technique I described for dealing with having to wake up at normal times despite my less than healthy sleep rhythm. Well, it was a good deal harder to do at that point in my life than when I was a young early twenty something, but I was still good to go if I got the right dose of Cotempla. Sure, I would crash at four in the afternoon, and crash hard, but at that point, I would be exhausted enough to just sleep for however long I needed to. I will be up by seven, no problem!

Oh, I was up by seven no problem, all right! See, I forgot that I did not actually have access to my pills when I put the plan in motion and would not until I went to stay at my parents. I managed to fight off the bone deep exhaustion with

McDonald's cokes and homebrewed coffee until my folks came to grab me and my graduation stuff, but I was quite desperate for my Cotempla hit by the time I got to my parents' estate so I would not feel like the walking dead any longer.

Sadly, this resulted in me intaking twice the amount I was prescribed. The dosage I took, when I searched online for what I should expect, Google said in big red letters and with official looking warning signs to call 911. Now!

I did as I was told. See, funny little mini story here. My Aunt Judy and Uncle Bob (Judy was the in-law) were also staying the night with my parents in preparation. They may have been staying there the whole week, but I cannot recall if that was the case. They had been there since at least the day before, as they were there to greet me early in the morning, and they were too cheery to have just gotten off a red-eye flight. My sister, Maren, was also staying there, but she was out at that point. Anyway, when I arrived, I greeted them and gave a darn good non-zombie performance (or at least, that is how I remember that). We exchanged pleasantries, before they went back up to their rooms to prepare for the day; the graduation was not until tomorrow, so they were prepping to go out and enjoy the pool and then get some breakfast. Immediately after they left was when I overdosed and called the paramedics. Imagine their shock when they came back down to enjoy the pool and some food, only to see the whole house swarming with every manner of first responder, from police to paramedics to firemen.

Luckily, they told me that beyond a high, even-for-me heart rate (which genuinely worried them until we told them my average heart rate; for a normal person, I was showing signs of having just survived a heart attack, and not merely the raised hear trate it was in my case) and some twitching, I was fine. I was to call if anything got worse though. They did tell me that there was no way I was getting to bed anytime soon. I was going to be riding this high for a few days yet.

When I fell asleep two days later, the feeling of relief was genuinely divine. Either that, or hellishly sinful. Either way, heaven or hell, it felt incredibly good when I finally fell asleep.

However, as I said, I was high on some powerful stimulants. From that point moving forwards, I took notes on how I felt, because if I ever wrote a book about zombies, this is how I would describe the "smart" superweapon zombies. The type used as an unkillable soldier and bioweapon, pitiless and single-minded as all zombies, but smart enough to use tools and advanced military tactics. The kind of zombie you gave a gun to. I felt like the living dead still, and yet I had all the alertness and articulation of someone who was fully awake. It was a bizarre contradiction of emotions, like a zombie who could think and use guns.

And so that is how, four o'clock the next morning, I was having breakfast at IHOP none the worse for wear to all eyes but my inner one. I had, quite frankly, too much food that morning. After I had my fill, I went to get everything paid for,

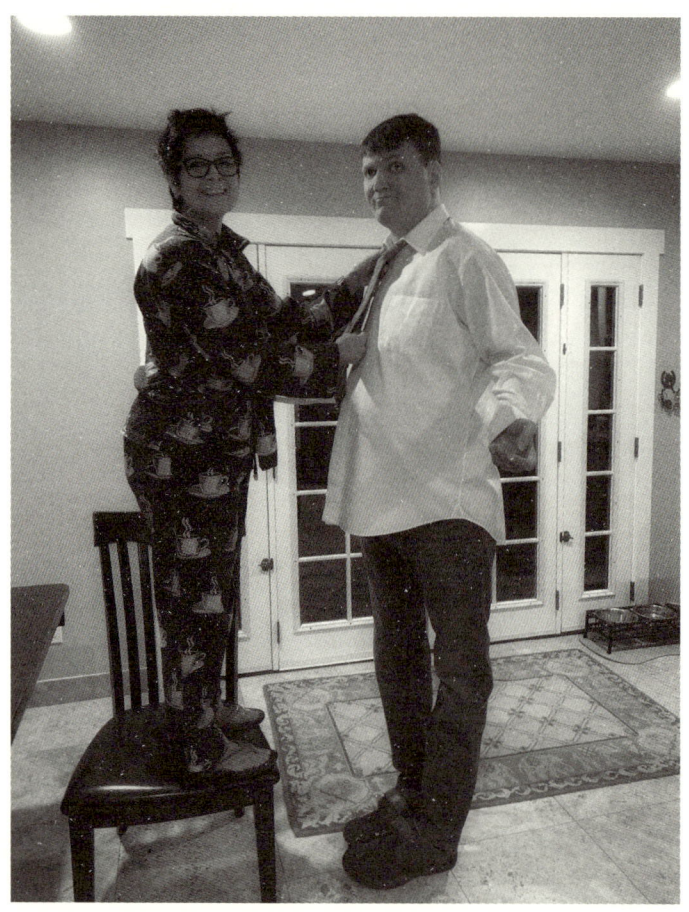

Graduating from ASU, I get some early morning sartorial help from my housemate and friend Liz Foldi.

when the last link in that chain of bizarre unfortunate events happened before the graduation proper. The cashier, a woman getting late in her years (probably in her seventies, if my guess is right), just froze. Then, she started to react to what I was saying in seemingly slow motion, as if God had hit the slow-motion button on her and her alone. You will have to forgive me and my still technically tired out mind/brain, but seeing as I had no experience in whatever this was, I genuinely thought I was witnessing proof of demonic possession being real or that simulation theory was correct and the computer running the universe was experiencing a glitch. This freaked me out enough to cause me to run out of the IHOP. Of course, I calmed downright quick when I realized that she still had my credit card in her frozen hands, and that she likely needed help.

I was going to call an ambulance (twice in a row), but at first I wanted to figure out if this was normal for her. So, I went in to ask around with the regulars and staff. Well, a group of old veterans (and I mean Vietnam War old when I say old) knew immediately what was going on; she was having a stroke.

Let me repeat; to crown the absolute surrealism of everything surrounding my graduation, my cashier at IHOP had a stroke in the middle of processing my payment.

I did not need to call the ambulance after all; the old vets called immediately after I talked to them. Another employee came out and accepted my payment and I headed back home just a touch more freaked out. Then graduation came, and surprise of all surprises, it went off without a hitch. No zombie plagues. The *Black Death* did not come back with a vengeance. There were no technical problems.

The whole thing was massively stupid; this was one of the largest graduating classes in the nation. There were a little more than a thousand graduates, including me. All the degrees were mailed because, even if we used a factory line, it would take too long for all of us to come on stage and grab a degree. When we were graduated, they called us out by major and graduated us altogether that way. They just told us to move our tassels and sit our butts down. Only those who were getting awards, who were valedictorians, or were for whatever reason warranted special mention went on that stage and got their degrees from the staff. It was my family that made the experience real and nothing that the school did to be honest:

> I was beside myself with emotion when you graduated from ASU. I knew how hard you fought to reach that accomplishment. Through the mental/physical challenges you did not let that stand in your way and you persevered. I will never forget your graduation day. I will admit I never walked for my graduation, so this was the first university graduation that I had attended. I remember walking into the stadium filled with soon-to-be graduates, professors, and families. I was immediately

moved to tears. I thought of all the times in the hospital and gaps you had to take to heal.... then you would start classes again and slowly chip away. You never gave up and kept your eye on the goal. I was so proud of my brother. (Maren Stuart)

Yet, beyond the truly odd sensation of being completely alert, despite having been up for about 50 hours by that point (dad jokingly told me that he doubted I was the only one high as a kite at that graduation; he was probably right) the graduation went on without event as was mentioned earlier.

Thus, I and a thousand other kids walked out of that repurposed stadium. Everyone else, sensing that this graduation was not all that traditional, decided not to toss their hats and keep them as a souvenir. Except for me. I had been stuck on that college hamster wheel far longer than I should have been, and I was finally done. Tossing that hat and losing track of the burgundy eyesore, never to see it again, really sealed the finality of it all. It was, to be clichéd, darn freeing! I never want to see that hat for the rest of my life! Not graduation caps in general; I am sure I will see plenty of those before the grave. Not, that hat.

I was still too high on Cotempla to sleep despite all that happened, the rest of the day passed till it was time to go to a five-star surf and turf restaurant in celebration. I enjoyed myself immensely, though I really wish I did not feel like a smart zombie for it.

On that note, the next day, I finally fell asleep. When I woke up, I met up with my parents and everyone else still staying there before they scattered throughout the country now that everything was done. I would be a writer! *Christopia* is open for business.

That is how this giraffe came to write this book. Or something like that!

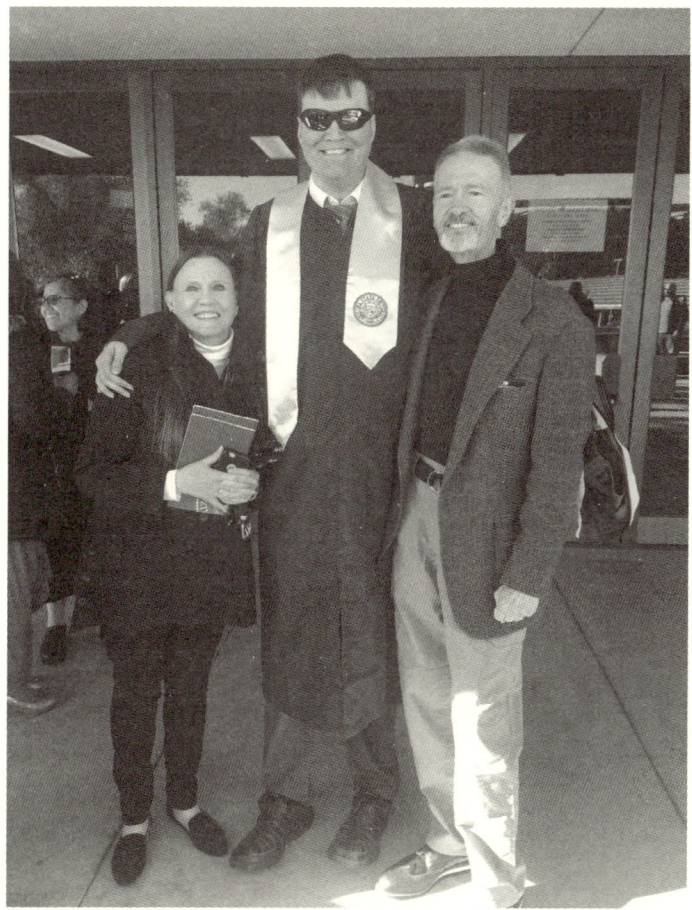
*Determined to graduate college before turning 30,
I beat my deadline by 3 weeks.*

DEDICATIONS

This last segment here was going to be something very different. It was going to be my concluding statements on this year-long journey, the journey of writing this book. I was going to give you, the parents, and you, my fellow kids (at heart) with Marfan syndrome, some advice. The best advice I could give in my own limited capacity and equally limited experience. It was going to be themed around that famous Frank Sinatra song "My Way"! All about how I rolled with, adapted to, flat out ignored all the punches life sent my way. I was going to tell all of you how you could do the same, hopefully.

But then, on the day I was typing out these last words, I received news that my mom, Ann Reinking, passed on. I knew what needed to be said here.

Do you want to know how, as parents, you can help your children with Marfan syndrome? Just follow my mom's example. She never gave up on me. She spared no expense nor love on me. She bled to find me the best care she could. Frankly, I literally would not be here typing this if she were not there for me. Firstly, because I would have almost certainly been dead, but also because she got me connected with The Marfan Foundation. She always supported them; I will continue to do so in her stead.

Simply follow the example of this remarkable woman; never ever give up.

In Loving Memory,
Ann Reinking
November 10, 1949—December 12, 2020

MARFAN SYNDROME

Marfan syndrome is a life-threatening genetic condition of the body's connective tissue. Knowing the signs of Marfan syndrome, getting a proper diagnosis, and receiving the necessary treatment can enable people with Marfan syndrome to live a long and full life.

About 1 in 5,000 people have Marfan syndrome. This includes men and women of all races and ethnic groups. Without proper diagnosis and treatment, they are at high risk for an early sudden death.

Some features of Marfan syndrome are easier to see than others. These include long arms, legs, and fingers; tall and thin body type; curved spine; sunken or protruding chest; flexible joints; flat feet; crowded teeth; and unexplained stretch marks on the skin.

Harder-to-detect signs include heart problems, especially related to the aorta, the large blood vessel that carries blood away from the heart. Additional features of Marfan are sudden collapse of a lung and eye problems, including severe nearsightedness, dislocated lens, detached retina, early glaucoma, and early cataracts.

Advances in medical care help people live longer and enjoy a good quality of life if they are diagnosed and treated. Most people with Marfan syndrome can work, go to school, and enjoy active hobbies. It is very important that people with Marfan syndrome get treatment and follow medical advice; otherwise, heart problems can cause sudden death. With an early diagnosis, helpful medical treatment can begin early in life.

THE MARFAN FOUNDATION

The Marfan Foundation's mission is to save lives and improve the quality of life of individuals with Marfan syndrome, Loeys-Dietz syndrome, Vascular Ehlers-Danlos syndrome, and other genetic aortic and vascular conditions. The Foundation, which was founded in 1981, tirelessly advances research for treatments that save lives and dramatically enhance quality of life for affected people and provides a supportive community for everyone affected by Marfan syndrome and related conditions. The Foundation always has the latest and most accurate information, and educates everyone—from individuals and families to medical professionals and the general public—about Marfan syndrome and related conditions.

FOR MORE INFORMATION, VISIT MARFAN.ORG.